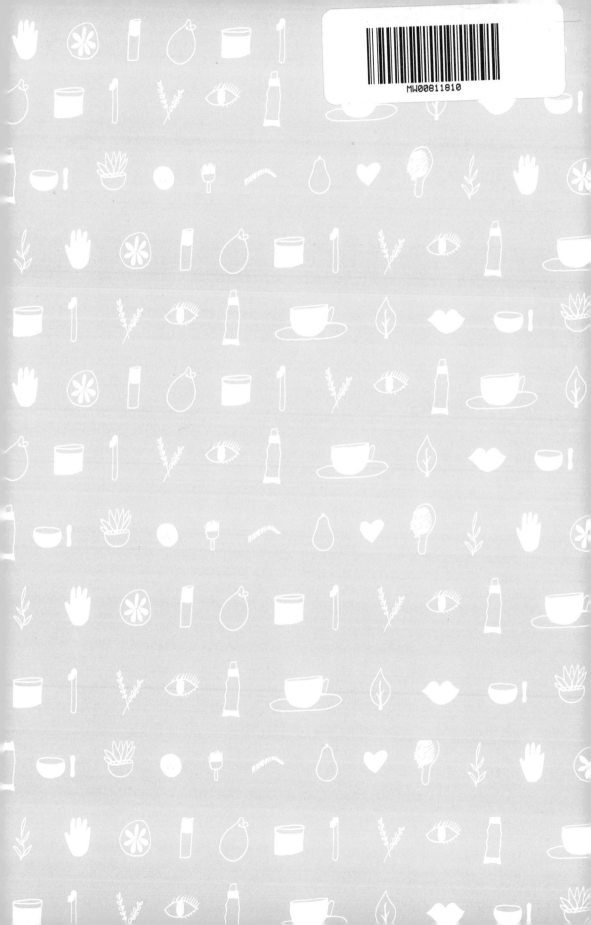

kalon (n.)
beauty that is more
than skin-deep.

DISCLAIMER

The contents of this book are for information only and are intended to assist readers in identifying symptoms and conditions they may be experiencing. This book is not intended to be a substitute for obtaining proper medical advice and must not be relied upon in this way. Always consult a qualified doctor or health practitioner. The author and publisher do not accept responsibility for illness arising out of the failure to seek medical advice from a doctor. In the event that you use any of the information in this book for yourself or your family or friends, the author and the publisher assume no responsibility for your actions.

The author and publisher have made every effort to ensure that the information in this book is correct at the time of printing and do not assume, and hereby disclaim, any liability to any party for any loss, damage, offence or disruption caused by errors or omissions, whether such errors or omissions result from negligence, accident, or any other cause.

Copyright © Dr Libby Weaver, 2018

Published by Little Green Frog Publishing Ltd

Publication design and illustrations:
Stephanie Antill. St. Clement Creative.

www.littlegreenfrogpublishing.com

ISBN: 978-0-473-43609-4

Printed in China

ALSO BY DR LIBBY WEAVER

Accidentally Overweight

Rushing Woman's Syndrome

Dr Libby's Real Food Chef, with Chef Cynthia Louise

Beauty from the Inside Out

Dr Libby's Real Food Kitchen, with Chef Cynthia Louise

The Calorie Fallacy

Sweet Food Story, with Chef Cynthia Louise

Exhausted to Energized

Women's Wellness Wisdom

The Energy Guide

What am I Supposed to Eat?

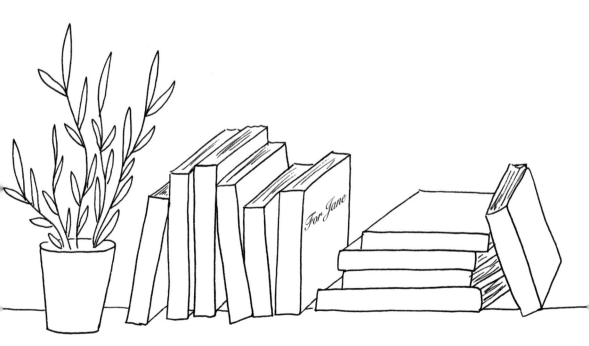

MY MISSION IS TO

EDUCATE & INSPIRE,

enhancing people's

HEALTH & HAPPINESS

Dr Libby Weaver

IGNITING A
RIPPLE EFFECT

~ *that* ~

transforms

THE WORLD.

–Dr Libby Weaver

CONTENTS

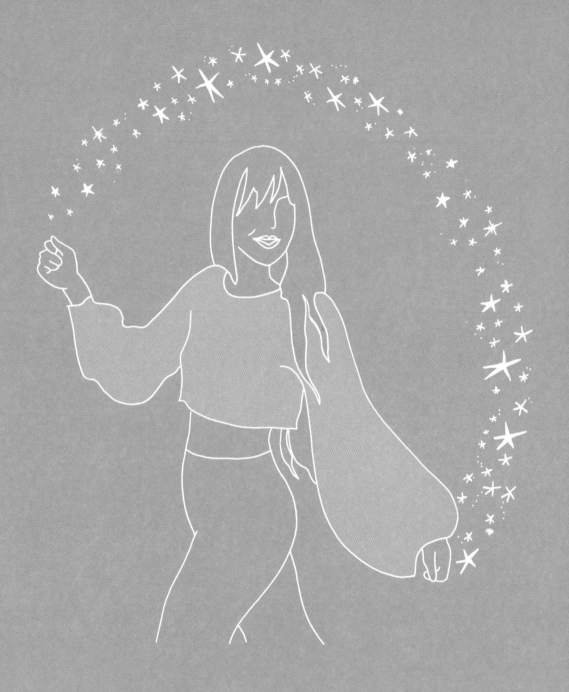

If you knew who you truly are,
you'd be in awe of yourself.

———

Introduction

The beauty you were born with

———

Not everyone cares about their health. On the one hand, this is unfathomable to me, yet on the other, I get it. If you've always had good health, if you've always been okay, if you've never experienced what it is like to try to exist (as opposed to 'live') without it, you don't know what you'll be missing out on in a state of poor health. Yet, in stark contrast, almost everyone cares about how they look. Some people actually use 'health' as a mask for wanting to look good.

For most people, it takes a health crisis, disease diagnosis or a debilitating decline in life quality before they truly learn that without our health, we have nothing. I don't want it to take that for you to start caring for yourself. I want to get you back in touch with how truly miraculous your body is and to care enough about yourself and the gift that is your life to act on that caring. I want you to notice your body's magnificent ability to draw your attention to the signs it gives you, and for you to have the tools to be able to decipher what those signs mean and then act to better support your body. And that's what this book is about. It's about helping you to understand what your body means when it gives you, for

example, skin challenges, and for you to be living so in touch with how precious you are that you treat your Earth Suit (what I lovingly call the body!) accordingly.

A REFLECTION OF INNER PROCESSES

Understanding that your skin, hair and nails, for example, are an exterior demonstration of what is going on inside you helps you to know where to begin if you'd like to make changes. Or, to put it in another way, what to do if your body is asking you to make changes by giving you certain signs that you may not welcome. Treat yourself with the love and compassion you deserve and see challenges in these areas, not as stumbling blocks that interfere with your joy in life, but rather as the guiding light that they are.

These days it is possible to obtain 'fake' versions of beauty bits that we may not be satisfied with. If we are dissatisfied with our nails, for example, it is common for people to get acrylic covers. There is absolutely nothing wrong with this. It can be fun and bring you great pleasure, so by all means do it. Yet I cannot encourage you enough to also work on your nail health from the inside out. Your nails can be a reflection of numerous interior processes, including nutritional status, protein metabolism and bone health. If these issues aren't addressed, my concern is that more significant health challenges could become apparent in the future.

If your hair is thinning, you can get hair extensions. However, you will benefit immensely if you work out why you are losing excessive amounts of hair (refer to the Hair help article on page 75). If the outer third of your eyebrow hair starts to fall out, you can choose to have them tattooed. Yet this hair loss can indicate that your thyroid needs support or that you are iron deficient. Both issues, if left untreated, can lead to far more major health consequences down the track.

So, by all means enjoy beauty salon nails, hair extensions or brow tattoos, but also focus on supporting the interior processes that these exterior signs might be highlighting. I hope this books helps you to do this. Deciphering challenges with beauty bits can light the way to better health.

Throughout this book I will be asking you to consider whether the parts of your body that sadden or frustrate you are simply messengers asking you to eat, drink, move, think, breathe, believe or perceive in a new way. See them as the gifts that they are, opening you to

a new way of living, learning and deeply appreciating who you are and your life. You'll notice I can't help but reiterate this concept, reminding you of the wisdom of your body and prompting you to question which one of these (or a number of these) may need attention. Is it your drinking, for example, or your perception of something or someone that needs to shift?

SEE YOUR BODY'S MESSAGES AS THE GIFTS THAT THEY ARE, OPENING YOU TO A NEW WAY OF LIVING, LEARNING AND DEEPLY APPRECIATING WHO YOU ARE AND YOUR LIFE.

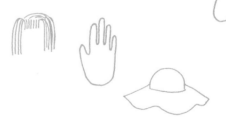

GENTLE AWE

If you knew who you truly are, you'd be in awe of yourself. Yet most people live their lives so out of touch with that. If you lived more in touch with the miracle that you are you probably wouldn't choose half the things you do. You also wouldn't feel like you need to fix or hide your true self.

Picture this. Imagine yourself as a baby. Perhaps you have a photo of yourself that captures a particular moment or maybe you simply remember. See that in your mind's eye. If you are struggling with how you perceive yourself today, it can sometimes help to remember that before anything actually happened in your life, you were a precious being. You didn't have to instruct yourself to start to grow up. Your body had an instinctual knowledge about what to do that is perfect for your journey. What power! Just in the same way a human doesn't have to tell a rosebud to open and become a rose, everything in nature, us included, has an innate wisdom within that fosters our beautiful selves to grow and become who we are.

Think of yourself when you were a baby again. Now picture yourself as a two-year-old. Notice the light in your eyes, your energy and playfulness and that you are growing up knowing in every fibre of your being that you are wonderful.

Now off you go to school—try to conjure a mental image of a photo from that time—are you still your bright-light self?

Or somewhere around that time did the light dim, even just slightly? I hope not, but for many, things start to change somewhere between four and seven years of age. You start to believe what you hear other people saying about you. You start to create meanings from the looks on people's faces about who you must be to be on the receiving end of those expressions and words— whether those words were harsh or just thoughtless throwaway comments that no one else noticed. And you start to doubt, for the very first time, thinking that maybe you aren't all that wonderful, or special, or precious, or lovable or worthy. Not consciously. You don't tend to sit around wondering and literally asking yourself those questions, but somewhere on the inside you start to question who you are and if you are loved.

You can't see, at this stage, that the people in your life are the way they are because of their joys and pains up until this point in time. You don't have that level of psychological maturity yet. The only way you can begin to make sense of what is going on is to create a belief in your own deficiency. You unknowingly start to believe—and act— as if something is wrong with you. You start to perceive flaws in yourself for the first time during this time: 'My nose is too big and so are my thighs', 'My clothes are old-fashioned and I'm so embarrassed'. And to feel safe, you do whatever you can to fit in. You want to be the same as everyone else, but you also want to stand out and be different. This is often exacerbated through our teenage years. And underneath it all, you are usually (unknowingly) trying to replace the love you perceive you've lost.

If you reflect on your choices across this period of growing up, some of what you will have chosen will have been due to trying to 'cover up' these perceived flaws. Perhaps you started not wanting to be seen outside your home without wearing layers of makeup, or you started smoking or started thinking about getting surgery to change aspects of your appearance. You will also have been trying to return to the state—the way of feeling—you had before you caught a glimpse of these perceived 'flaws', trying to return to being the precious, beautiful soul that you are (but no longer believe yourself to be). It is very confusing as you usually have friends across this time in your life who you can tell like you. But somewhere inside yourself, you don't really like or appreciate yourself any more. And your choices reflect this.

If you look back at this time in your life— or perhaps you are going through it while you are reading this—it tended to be a time of uncertainty and confusion. A time when you felt awkward and embarrassed regularly. There may have been periods where you felt ashamed or shameful of yourself, but you couldn't really articulate that this is how you felt; your behaviour just tended to be quiet and withdrawn or angry and snappy. You heard any feedback or comments as criticism and whether you showed it or not, this hurt your heart. You were/are terrified of failure and rejection.

Yet when you pause to reflect on this period of your past, ask yourself: how did someone as wonderful and precious and adorable and special and lovable as you end up so demoralised, dispirited, disheartened, disempowered? For that precious soul, with all of that innate knowing and wisdom and power, is still inside you. It is still who you are. And I hope this book helps you to return to the truth of who you are, what you were born knowing: that you are wonderful and special and important and so very beautiful ∎

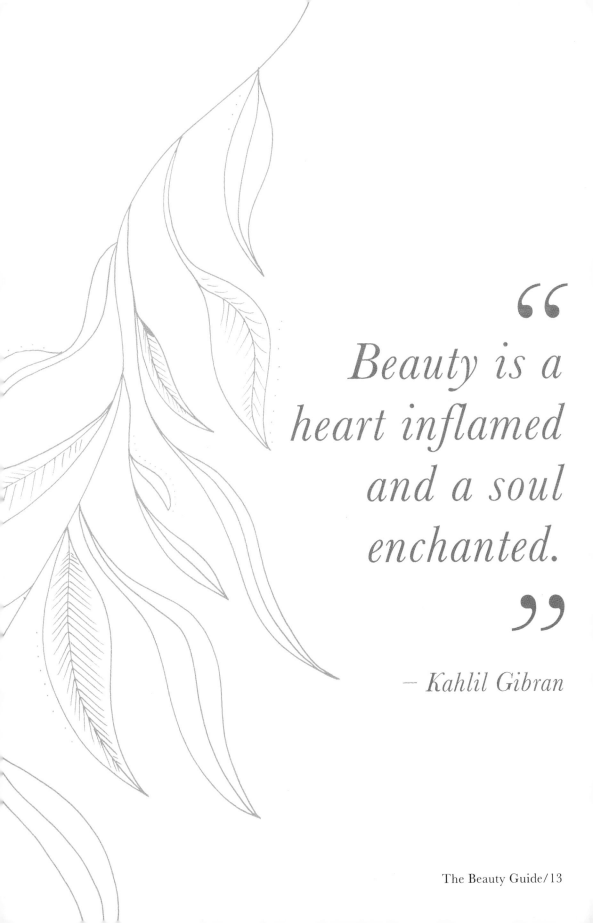

“

Beauty is a heart inflamed and a soul enchanted.

”

— *Kahlil Gibran*

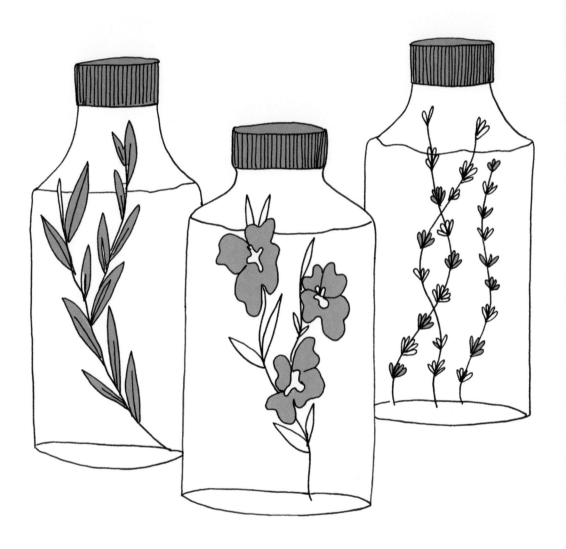

Dr Libby Weaver

The foundation

Beauty from the inside out

There are three lenses through which we shall explore your health and what I refer to as the beauty bits: the outer parts of our body that we can see which most attribute to physical beauty such as the skin, hair and nails. Those three lenses are the pillars of my work, the way I examine everything, and they are:

1. the biochemical
2. the nutritional
3. the emotional.

For great health and sparkle you want to understand all three pillars and this book offers you that. For now, however, let's start at the beginning and understand what is required for your body to create inner health and outer vitality.

BEAUTY FROM THE INSIDE OUT

The amount of time, focus and money spent on trying to sort out exterior problems that are actually created from inside processes gone awry is astronomical. Every cell of your body (and there are about 50 trillion of them), not just skin cells on the outside, contributes to how you feel and look every minute of every day. And those cells need both nutrients and efficient waste-removal systems for you to feel and look your best.

The biochemical pathways of your body also need to work efficiently and, to do this, nutrients are required. So, what is a biochemical reaction? It is where one substance is converted into another substance. That is one reaction. Then that new substance will be converted into something else in another reaction. Every second, there are billions of biochemical reactions occurring inside you. Doesn't that blow your mind?

For each reaction, a nutrient or a number of nutrients are required. That means, if we become nutritionally deficient, the efficiency of our body to change one substance into something else can become compromised. As a result we suffer on the inside (think bloated tummy) or on the outside (think congested skin).

To ensure that the biochemistry of our inner world is giving us what we want on the outside—great energy and clear skin jump to mind for many—we need to ensure that we are providing ourselves with the nutrients needed for these reactions and to nourish every cell. But this is only half the picture. We also need to ensure that the waste-disposal systems of the cells and the overall body are working at their best.

Let's explore how we can do this ■

Beauty nourishment

What goes in and what goes out

Vitamins and minerals are needed to drive almost all of the biochemical reactions in your body that determine how you feel, function and look. So we want to ensure the reactions are getting what they need! Nutrients are also needed to nourish every cell of your body, and you are essentially the result of the health of your cells. What this means is that if the needs of the cell aren't met, there are consequences with how you look or how you feel—or both.

The only way you obtain nutrients is through what you eat, which is one major reason why you'll hear me remind you of the vital importance of eating whole, real food and minimising (or omitting) processed foods. You want maximum nourishment and nutrient density rather than artificial and poor-quality non-food. Think 'nourishment' with as many mouthfuls as possible.

What is just as important to the nourishment of a cell is its ability to get rid of waste. In the same way as you, as a whole human, eliminate your waste, each cell eats and then disposes of excrement. Cellular waste ends up in the lymphatic fluid. This doesn't have a pump to get it moving away from where the waste was deposited and, for it to function at its best, you don't want waste accumulating around the cell. Blood has a pump—the heart—but lymphatic fluid only moves when we move. Its motion is stimulated by diaphragmatic breathing, bouncing on a trampoline, walking, yoga, Pilates, tai chi and massage. Some medicinal herbs, such as St Mary's thistle, can also help to support the lymphatic system, by promoting detoxification of cellular waste.

THE ONLY WAY YOU OBTAIN NUTRIENTS IS THROUGH WHAT YOU EAT.

The more efficient your body is at obtaining nutrients (you impact this by what you eat), absorbing nutrients (refer to the information about digestion on page 93 for more on this) and eliminating waste, both from around the local cellular environment and from the human body as a whole, the more you will look and feel your best. I hope the information in this book helps you do all three of these vital processes exceptionally well so you have outstanding health and radiance ■

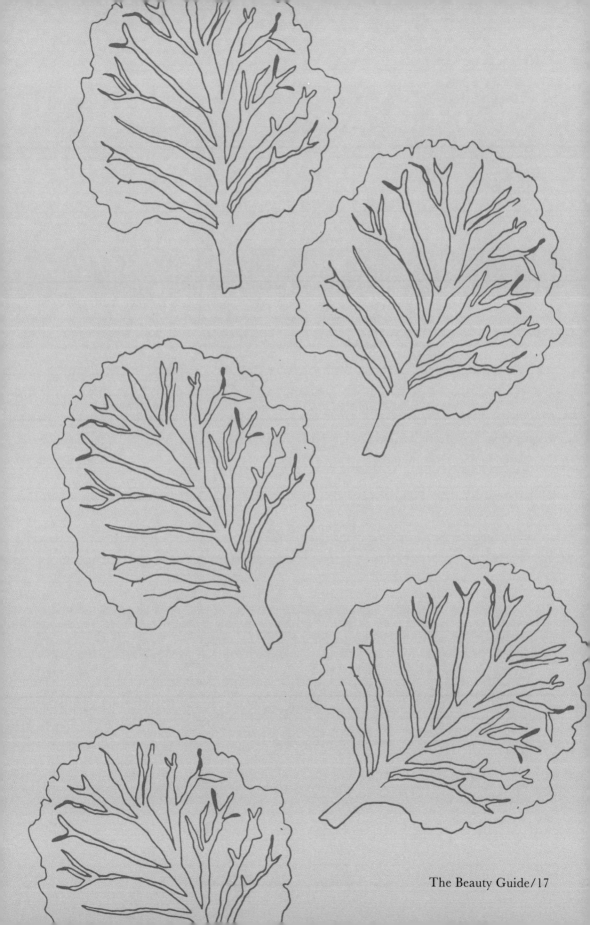

TIME

LESS
beauty

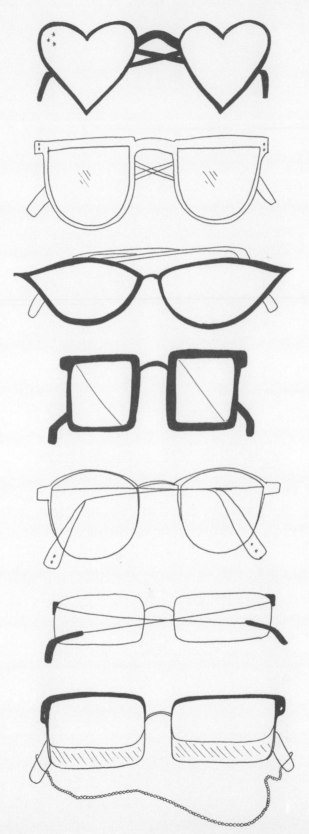

Dr Libby Weaver

Understanding ageing

A graceful transition

Ageing is *supposed* to happen. We can't escape it or deny it. However, the level of debilitation it can cause or the speed at which it happens is something we can influence through our daily choices, particularly by what we eat and our perception of what constitutes stress. Not only do stress hormones have their own ageing actions via their ability to break down muscle, but the stress response typically increases breathing rates, which as you'll see can increase the substances that age us from the inside out.

THE THREE MAIN WAYS WE AGE ARE:

1. oxidation
2. inflammation
3. glycation.

All of these processes can be damaging in themselves. Plus, they can have a detrimental impact on telomeres, which are structures at the end of our chromosomes that play a role in protecting our genetic information.

Let's understand this more and work out simple steps that can help us to prevent these degenerative processes from happening too quickly.

OXIDATION:

Also known as oxidative stress, this is one of the major causes of ageing. Damage is done to our DNA, body proteins and fats by free radicals, single fragmented oxygen units (we're talking of the molecular level here) who aren't happy because oxygen likes to be stuck together with another unit of oxygen. Free radicals are produced when we breathe and a small number of them help the body with some vital processes, such as helping us get over an infection. However, when they are in excessive numbers, degeneration (ageing) occurs. Free radicals are also produced during inflammatory reactions and as a result of exposure to, or consumption of, pollutants. Cigarettes, for example, accelerate ageing in this way (as well as in other ways). To help protect ourselves from the damage that free radicals have the potential to cause, we need to consume antioxidant-rich foods (found predominantly in coloured plant foods) as these foods can donate an oxygen unit back to the single grumpy guy. Paired back up with his buddy, he is as happy as a duck and will no longer damage your tissues.

There is more to consider here. What leads you to turn over more oxygen? In other words, what leads you to breathe more rapidly? Cardiovascular exercise and stress are two causes. More rapid breathing leads to more free-radical production, which requires more antioxidants to be consumed in order to avoid excessive damage. Consider this: during the cardiovascular exercise craze of the 80s and 90s, were people advised to eat more antioxidants? No! Nutritionally, that era predominantly focused on eating low-fat foods! Yet without the simultaneous increase in antioxidant-rich foods alongside all of that cardio, ageing processes get accelerated. Moral of the story? Eat your vegies, everyone!

And so, what about stress? When you are stressed, do you tend to eat better or worse than usual? Usually worse; right when you need to be eating better! This is one reason why some people will say that they feel (or look) like they've aged rapidly after a stressful time.

INFLAMMATION:

Inflammation is another way we age. We associate inflammation with heat, redness and swelling, and sometimes these signs are visible on the skin. Eczema, for example, has inflammatory aspects to it (as well as immune aspects), yet there can also be inflammation occurring on the inside, hidden from our view.

Put simply, inflammation is one of the ways your immune system responds to a substance it deems problematic entering your body. How do things enter? You can ingest them, breathe them, or you can absorb them through your skin.

When your immune system perceives that a threatening substance has entered, it mounts a powerful and multi-pronged attack on the 'invader'. Part of that response is to create inflammation (the heat, swelling and redness), which occurs wherever the immune system is engaged in a battle—in the tissues of your face, in your blood vessels, and/or in your vital organs, for example. Inflammation is essential to keeping us alive, but it also causes collateral damage, such as scarring and wrinkling.

Do what you can to minimise your exposure to pollutants and support the detoxification and elimination pathways of the body to get rid of the things we can't help but take in (explained in more detail on page 88).

GLYCATION:

Another factor that contributes to ageing is glycation. This occurs when glucose, fructose or galactose (sugars) from what we eat bind to some of our DNA, proteins and lipids (fats), leaving them unable to do their jobs. The by-product of this is what are known as advanced glycation end products (AGEs). If we have a diet high in processed and deep-fried foods, the problem becomes worse as we get older, since the cumulative sugar intake for most just keeps growing. This can cause cells and tissues to not work properly, resulting in ageing or, in some cases, disease.

Not that long ago in human evolution, processed high-sugar foods didn't exist. Then, in the not-so-distant past, they were eaten only on special occasions, such as birthday parties. Now, however, they are a part of every day for too many people. I cannot say this enough: it is what you do every day that impacts on your health, not what you do sometimes. The ageing process will potentially be slowed if you consume fewer high-sugar, processed and deep-fried foods.

TELOMERES:

Our genes are located on twisted, double-stranded molecules of DNA called chromosomes inside the centre (nucleus) of cells. Structures called telomeres protect our genetic information. Their protective capacity allows cells to divide successfully and replace old cells with (ideally) good-quality new cells. In many textbooks, telomeres have been compared with the plastic tips on shoelaces because they prevent chromosome ends from fraying and sticking to each other, which would scramble our genetic data and possibly lead to disease or death (1). However, each time a cell divides, the telomeres get shorter. When they get too short, the cell can no longer replicate itself and it becomes inactive or dies. This is one of the processes associated with ageing.

An enzyme named telomerase adds structures (called bases) to the ends of telomeres to help counteract their shortening. In young cells, telomerase keeps telomeres from being worn down too much. But as cells divide repeatedly, there is not enough telomerase, so the telomeres grow shorter and the cells age (1). While telomere shortening has been linked to the ageing process, scientists have not yet deciphered whether shorter telomeres are just a sign of ageing (like grey hair) or actually contribute to ageing (1). What we are starting to understand, however, is that antioxidants potentially play a role in slowing telomere shortening. Yet another reason why amping up your antioxidant consumption (read, vegetables!) needs to be high on your priority list ■

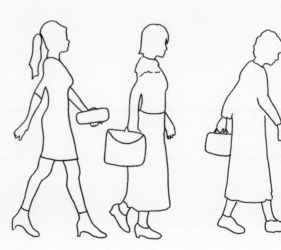

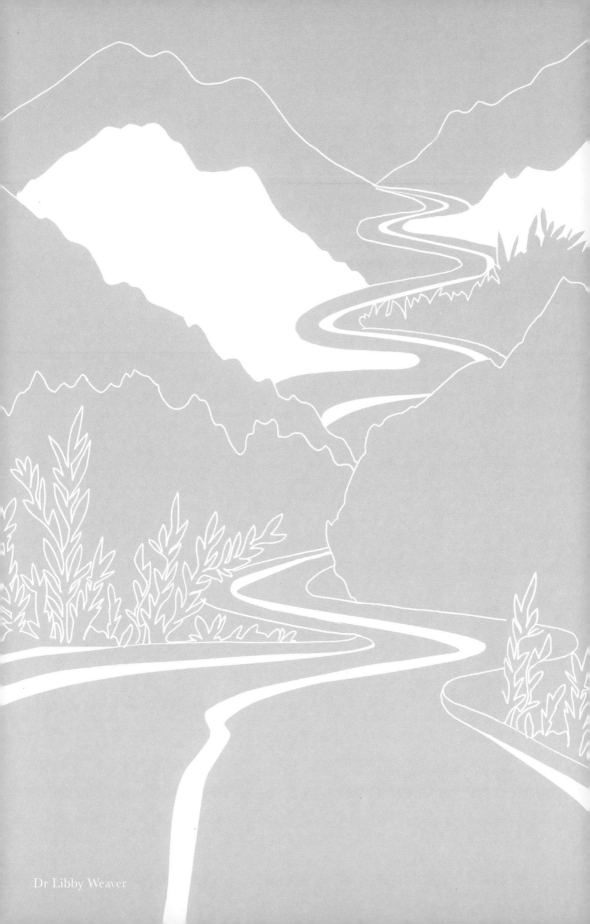

Dr Libby Weaver

The quality of your life

Are we living too short and dying too long?

———

We are fortunate to be living at a time where life expectancy is getting longer and longer, although trends suggest this may not continue for much longer in some countries, such as the US. We are so very fortunate to have access to extraordinary emergency medicine for accidents and other life-threatening situations. However, many people don't find themselves in these dire scenarios. Rather, they slowly find that their quality of life is deteriorating. It is this quality of your life that I care so much about.

To that end, a great question to ponder is: are we living too short and dying too long?

Both now and in the second half of your life, you want to be able to bend over and do up your own shoelaces. Imagine losing that level of independence and relying on someone else to tend to such a basic need. How would that feel?

We don't often pause to think about what life would be like if we lost the strength or flexibility of our bodies and could no longer do such tasks for ourselves. Sadly, it usually takes for this to be taken away before we even think about how great it was when we could put our own shoes on. When you meet people in this situation they often regret some of the choices they made around their health in the first half of their life very much.

You don't want your tummy to get so big that you can no longer do up your shoes. Also, you don't want to have been so thin earlier in your life with very little muscle mass that your bone density is now so low that you can't put your shoes on because your bones are so damaged and fragile. You don't want your spine to have become so inflexible from leading such a sedentary lifestyle that you can no longer reach your toes.

———

THE CHOICES YOU MAKE TODAY DON'T JUST INFLUENCE WHAT YOUR LIFE LOOKS LIKE NOW, THEY ARE GOING TO IMPACT YOUR ENTIRE FUTURE.

———

The power to change that is in your hands and in your hands only. No one can do it for you. But here's the kicker, and this is the part that is the biggest challenge for most people. You have to care enough about yourself to do this. Too many people believe deep down that they are worthless, or unworthy of care, which is one reason why so many people put their own health lower on their priority list than meeting the needs of work or family. Both of which, of course, are incredibly important, but both of which will suffer if you lose your health.

Also consider how you see yourself and the way you speak to yourself within this context of diminishing your quality of life. Are your judgements of your appearance or on aspects of your personality harsh? And are you harsh on others as a result? What do you say about yourself, to yourself? Is it kind, thoughtful, supportive and encouraging most of the time? Or the opposite? When you sit back and reflect at the end of your life (if you get the opportunity to do so) will you feel good about the way you spoke to yourself? Imagine all of the energy you waste putting yourself down that could be put to better use.

TRUSTING YOURSELF

DAILY HYDRATION

A GRATEFUL HEART

OWNING MINIMAL ITEMS OR LIVING SIMPLY

SHARING YOUR GIFTS WITH THE WORLD

NUTRIENTS,
ANTIOXIDANTS AND
PHYTOCHEMICALS
FROM WHOLE,
REAL FOODS

GOOD-QUALITY,
RESTFUL SLEEP

BEING
AUTHENTICALLY
YOU

What do you need to have a great quality life now and in the future? What allows you to live a beautiful life?

Here are some ideas to start you off.

LOVING YOUR
DEAR SELF

NO OR VERY
LITTLE
REFINED
SUGAR

GREAT
ENERGY

MINIMAL
LIVER LOADERS
(see page 90 for
more on this)

APPRECIATING
NATURE

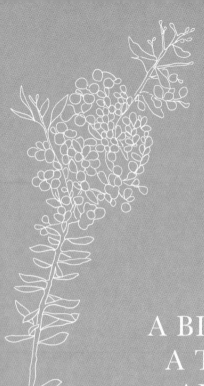

"

A BIRD SITTING ON
A TREE IS NEVER
AFRAID OF THE
BRANCH BREAKING,
BECAUSE HER TRUST
IS NOT IN THE
BRANCH BUT IN HER
OWN WINGS. ALWAYS
BELIEVE IN YOURSELF.

"

— *Anonymous*

Q
WHAT WOULD YOU INCLUDE IN YOUR LIST, OR WHAT WOULD YOU ADD TO THIS LIST?

I also want you to see that the outside falls into place when we act on experiencing a great quality life and taking care of our body, mind and soul. Your inner fire lights up your face as well as being a light in the world. If some of the ideas on page 27 resonate for you, consider how you will act on them and note this here.

For example, if for you, having great energy is a necessary part of you leading a great quality, beautiful life, you might write:

Q: What do I need?

A: Great energy.

Q: How will I do/create this?

A: I will eat real foods and make water my main drink. I will get 8 hours sleep most nights of the week. I will say no when I need to. I will schedule my tasks and time more so that I'm not doing everything at the last minute. I won't sweat the small stuff.

If you notice that your quality of life is reduced or that you feel like you unravel when you have too much on your plate—and that this ages you more than anything—instead of trying to work out how to make ends meet, work on having fewer ends (1).

Q: What do I need?

A: A simpler life.

Q: How will I create this?

A: Eat whole, real food for great brain (and body) function to begin to solve this. Less (or no) caffeine so I remain calm and have clarity of thought. I will prioritise my sleep for the above reasons, too. I will work out what my values are and live them. Spend more time in nature. Make a list of what I spend my money on and work out what I can let go of. Walk more, drive less. Stop comparing myself to others. Live life in touch with the fact that I am enough and that I therefore have enough ■

Your turn.

What does a *GREAT-* QUALITY LIFE look like for you?

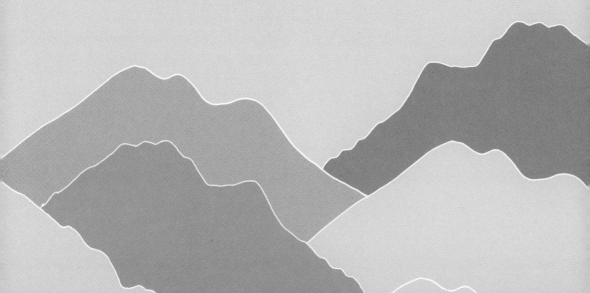

A:

“

Are you

TOO YOUNG *TO FEEL* AS OLD

as you do? ”

Dr Libby Weaver

The beauty of energy

Spark up that inner radiance

When you have great energy, it impacts so many of our choices in a wonderful way, as well as the sparkle in our eyes.

When you come into contact with someone who radiates great energy, what happens to you? You are uplifted, aren't you? Having great energy is a win-win for all involved!

When you have great energy, it is like you are lit up from inside. This doesn't just help you but encourages others to do the same. Become conscious of all of the tiny decisions across your day that essentially make up your health and energy. Make even more choices that continue to foster that light.

Energy does not have to decline as we age, taking its toll on our quality of life as it happens. Work on making choices that foster great energy across your whole life. For if we are tired it impacts the food that we choose, whether we get off the couch and go for a walk or not, friends that we make, jobs we have the confidence to apply for, our self-talk and the way we speak to everyone we love.

IF YOU DON'T HAVE GREAT ENERGY, WHAT IS CONTRIBUTING TO THAT?

Is it:

- poor quality food choices
- too much caffeine
- too much alcohol
- dehydration
- low muscle mass
- not enough hours spent in bed
- poor-quality sleep—unrefreshed upon waking despite spending enough hours in bed
- too much time spent sitting
- too many tabs open in your mind
- saying yes when you really want to say no
- feeling overwhelmed?

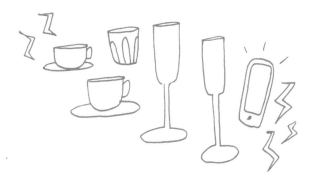

Energy is the true currency of health. For too long the way women (and men, but not in quite the same way) have assessed themselves is via their weight. When you weigh yourself, all you weigh is your self-esteem. You might not necessarily think this, but imagine if you kept weighing yourself to discover that no matter how hard you'd been trying, your weight kept increasing. Would you feel deflated or uplifted by this? Would it help you feel good about yourself?

The feminine essence responds to praise (the masculine to challenge) so when a female is not the weight she wants to be, it gives rise to a sense of deflation and failure, and it scratches the itch that she is still not good (in this case, slim) enough. Starting the day in this way does not uplift, inspire and energise you to take great care of yourself across the day. Shift your focus to making choices that better support your energy rather than your weight or body size. And watch the latter fall into place without deprivation or dieting, while your quality of life is enhanced through better energy.

Think of it like this: we are born with a certain amount of energy and from that moment forward we are either making choices (with what we eat, drink or via the thoughts that we think) that enhance our energy or take away from it. You can see your energy like a bank account. You are either making deposits into or withdrawals out of the account with each choice. Too many people predominantly make withdrawals across their days and nights, week after week, year after year. And after living too long like this, you end up living in overdraft. And to keep this analogy going, you then pay interest on that overdraft in the form of health and visible ('outer beauty') consequences.

THINK OF IT LIKE THIS: WE ARE BORN WITH A CERTAIN AMOUNT OF ENERGY AND FROM THAT MOMENT FORWARD WE ARE EITHER MAKING CHOICES THAT ENHANCE OUR ENERGY OR TAKE AWAY FROM IT.

What does withdrawing from your energy account look like? It looks like relying on caffeine to provide you with energy, eating poor-quality, processed, sweet food to try to get yourself through the afternoon, walking around with more open than closed loops, too much screen time, allowing yourself to be affected by things that are beyond your control, going to bed too late night after night, year after year, continuing to say yes to things when you know in your heart that your energy would benefit by creating even just a small amount of space for you.

This is not an all or nothing concept. It doesn't mean you need to stop making all withdrawals. It would be highly beneficial for you to make fewer of them, but most people find it easier to implement the concept of simply making more deposits into their energy bank account. And slowly but surely the energy scales start to tip in the direction of you feeling—and looking—better as a result.

WHAT FORM WILL YOUR ENERGY DEPOSITS TAKE?

Note them down. Here are some ideas to get you started.

Don't forget the power of whole, real food, including plenty of plants. Yes, that means vegetables! There is so much power in a nutrient-dense way of eating. When we're focused on eating to maintain (or change) our body shape and size, we tend to think about eating less; we might be focused on calorie intake versus energy we burn—the calorie equation. But no amount of exercise can work off a lousy way of eating. I can't emphasise enough the importance of prioritising a nourishing way of eating. While our macronutrients (protein, fats and carbs) provide us with energy (measured in calories or kilojoules), it is the micronutrients (vitamins and minerals) that allow us to extract and experience this energy. And whole, real foods contain both.

Work on closing what I call 'open tabs'. These are tasks, emails or jobs that haven't been resolved. It's as if we walk around each day with so many tabs open in our brains—like tabs sitting on your computer or phone. It's no wonder we feel drained and flattened!

Incorporate more resistance training or muscle-building exercise. This helps to build muscle mass. More muscle means more energy-producing mitochondria in our cells resulting in a higher metabolic rate, which assists with body fat management as well as energy production. Naturally, you gain better energy reserves as your glycogen (glucose stores) increase, as well.

Explore your perceptions. Be conscious of how your perceptions influence your mood and energy state. Write a list of what makes you feel alive and energised, and what saps your energy—your 'energy vampires'. Actively work on doing more of the things that make you feel energised while simultaneously reducing your energy vampires.

Let yourself have what you already have. When we live most moments in the pursuit of achievement, or of obtaining something, we are not focused on what is already in our lives. When you speak to people who are dying and you ask them what they are going to miss most in this word, they tell you the most ordinary things: their partner's face, their dog's fur, the smell of a freshly cut lemon, the night sky. We have all of that right now. So why not let yourself have what you already have, for it is what joy is all about and joy gives us an irreplaceable depth of energy ∎

Your turn…

Q WHAT MAKES YOU FEEL ALIVE AND FULL OF VITALITY?

A:

_____

_____

_____

_____

_____

Q: WHAT ARE YOUR 'ENERGY VAMPIRES'?

A:

_____

_____

_____

Q: WHAT DO YOU CURRENTLY DO TO ADD TO YOUR ENERGY ACCOUNT?

A:

_____

_____

_____

_____

Dr Libby Weaver

Q: WHAT ARE THE CURRENT WITHDRAWALS FROM YOUR
ENERGY ACCOUNT?

A:

_____

_____

_____

_____

_____

Q: LIST THE WAYS YOU CAN REDUCE THESE WITHDRAWALS
OR INCREASE YOUR DEPOSITS.

A:

_____

_____

_____

_____

_____

_____

_____

_____

_____

Beauty sleep

What happens when we rest?

———

There is a reason it's called 'beauty sleep'. While we sleep, critical repair work goes on inside of us that happens at much more minimal rates during the day while we are active. Yet, far too many people today don't get enough sleep— either from a lack of hours in bed because they are busy doing other things and not prioritising sleep, or the hours they do get don't refresh them. They wake up just as tired as when they went to bed.

Sleep is supposed to be restorative. Yet, how many people wake up these days and bound out of bed, full of vitality, excited about the day ahead? For too many, the day begins with wondering how it can be morning already and pressing the snooze button a few times. Plus, the use of sleeping tablets has become rife across the Western world.

So what on earth is going on when our body has lost the ability to do something so basic, so essential and fundamental to our wellbeing? There are many reasons why people don't sleep well. A major one today is due to living in sympathetic nervous system (SNS) dominance all day. If your body believes that your life is in danger, the last thing it wants for you is to sleep deeply as it is concerned that you may not wake up in time to save your own life. Yet, if the elevated stress hormone production is due to psychological stress, it is not needed to fuel an escape, and remaining slightly awake only serves to take away from your energy and your body's ability to do its vital repair work— adding to the stress load on your body.

———

SLEEP, OR A LACK OF QUALITY, RESTORATIVE REST, CAN HAVE A SIGNIFICANT IMPACT ON HOW WE LOOK AND FEEL EACH DAY.

———

If you don't wake up refreshed, get to the heart of why this is and resolve it. Would a breath-focused practice 30 minutes before bed help you to feel more relaxed so you fall asleep easier? Light destroys melatonin, one of our sleep hormones. Therefore, maybe you need to try avoiding back-lit devices for two hours before bed. Your muscles need magnesium to relax, so adding more magnesium-rich foods to your day, such as green leafy vegies, nuts and seeds, may help. Adults need seven to nine hours of sleep per night. We cannot fight our biology.

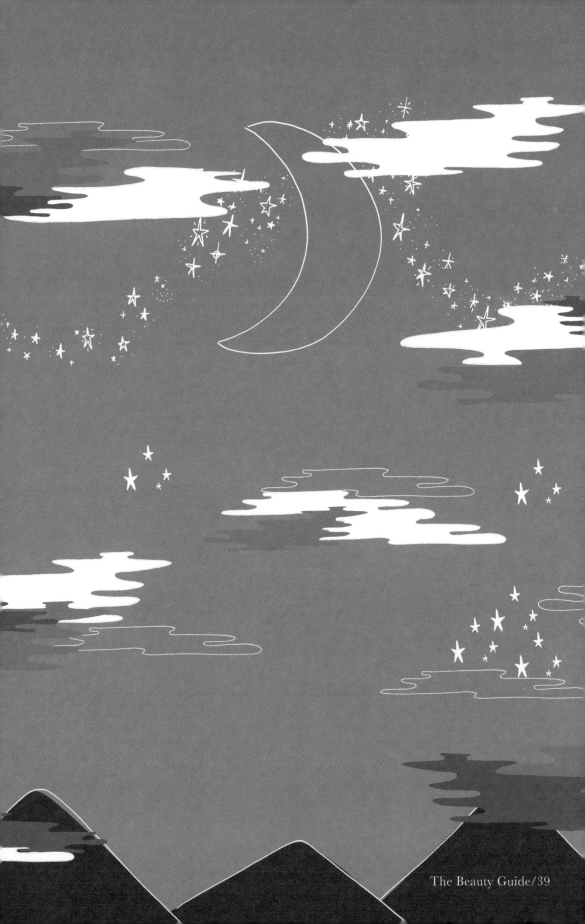

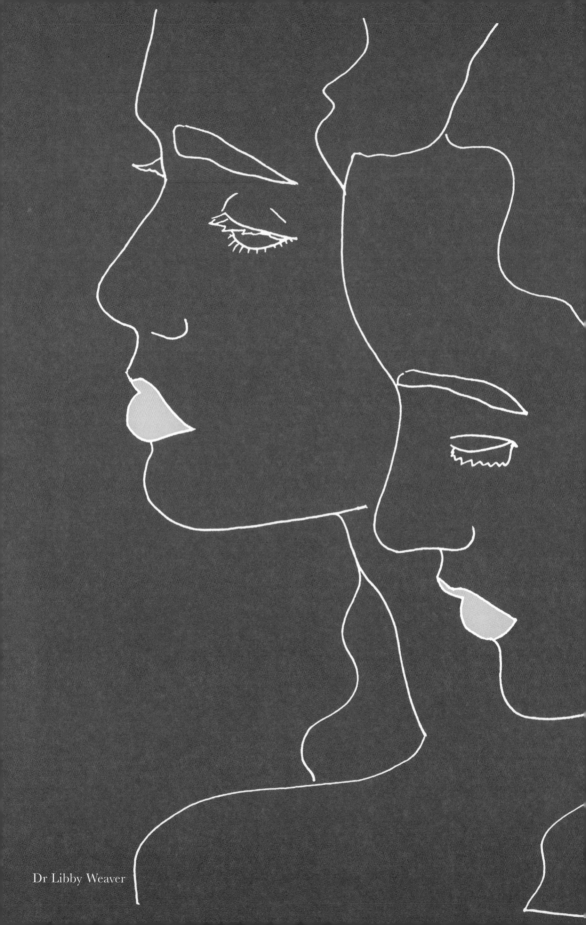

Dr Libby Weaver

The changing face of 40ish

Supporting your body as it ages

———

I could have picked any age really: 30, 40 or 50 and beyond. We notice changes at all ages, but it is often the zero years that have us honing in on what is different from years gone by. So, what happens around the age of 40 and what steps can we take to counteract some of what could unfold? Here are some of them.

The collagen and elastic fibres that keep skin smooth and youthful in appearance start to regenerate at a slower rate. This means more visible signs of ageing start to appear on the surface. This is partly due to the cumulative impact of damage done by free radicals, single oxygen units that damage tissues (refer to page 21 for more on these). It is also due to the repetition of facial expressions—you can see in the lines on people's faces if they have had decades of struggle and hardship or a more peaceful life. Regardless of which pattern predominates for you, seeing those lines as even more evidence of the extraordinary human you are helps you to accept them. In those lines you might see resilience, courage, resourcefulness, wisdom or happiness—or a whole plethora of other character traits.

Or it might be stretch marks. You may have had a child or children and now have stretch marks as a result of your miraculous body being able to grow and birth a child. In other words, your stretch marks are a visible sign of the miracle you are and that your baby is. Or you may have once had a bigger body size than you do now and stretch marks are evidence of a time gone by. Or a desire to overeat that you still find challenging. So, you see your stretch marks as a sign of your strength and determination and ongoing self-care.

———

NOTHING HAS MEANING IN THIS WORLD UNLESS WE GIVE IT MEANING.

———

The more uplifting meanings you attribute to these things, the more peace you will have and the more fuel you will have to take care of yourself, those you love and also to be able to share your gifts with the world.

Your forties can also be a time in your life when your menstrual cycle starts to change. The menstrual blood may become heavier, contain more clots and you may notice your mood becomes darker or harder to handle in the lead-up to your period. Perhaps your cycle shortens and where it was once 28 days, it's now more like 21. For others, their period becomes scarcer or scanty, less regular, the bleeding more infrequent. Perhaps you are starting to overheat easily or notice that your sleep has become more erratic and not refreshing.

As hormone levels change, it can also be a time when you notice changes in your body fat that can't be explained through how you eat and move, and perhaps this frustrates you. Some (not all) women notice a thickening of the torso around this time and there are a number of hormonal mechanisms behind this. It can be cortisol-related (refer to page 116) or due to estrogen levels dropping. As the ovaries cease to make sex hormones (estrogen and progesterone), the adrenal glands are supposed to continue to make a small amount of them.

When they do, you suffer much less through the transition into menopause. But for many women, their adrenals haven't made sex hormones for years or decades due to the constant, relentless output of stress hormones (refer to page 115). Body fat also makes estrogen so to compensate for poor adrenal health, the body responds (remembering your body always has your back!) by increasing your body fat so you can have some estrogen. There are two body systems in particular that typically need support in these scenarios: the liver and the adrenals, remembering that behind that is the 'am I safe?' scenario with the pituitary and the hypothalamus (refer to page 122).

At any age, a big life change can occur that we relish or find challenging. The longer you live, the more likely you are to have experienced these and suffered (though hopefully also grown) as a result. It might be the passing of someone close to you. A parent perhaps, or a dear friend. It might be the end of a major relationship or a pile of things all happening at once such as moving house, a sick child, too much work on your plate and an unrelenting sense of being overwhelmed because you feel like you have to deal with everything by yourself.

Your mantra may have become 'if I don't do it, it won't get done'. And if you tune in to how your body feels when you recite this, it hardens you, right when you need more softness and fluidity for the health of your body, mind and soul. This can also be a time when you feel a heavy burden of responsibility in many areas of your life and you start to wonder: 'When is it going to be my turn? When will I get to do more of what I want to do?' Feeling like this is a guide for you to start to identify what those things are and to begin to work out ways to bring more of them in to your life.

Regardless of your current age, here are some suggestions that can help to address some of the things discussed above and help you to transition through the years with ease and grace.

CHANGES TO YOUR SKIN

To address lines in your skin and reduce the appearance of stretch marks, minimise free radical damage by consuming a diet rich in coloured plant foods which are high in antioxidants. You may like to take additional vitamin C. Don't smoke and do what you can to avoid exposure to pollutants and other problematic substances. Support your body to eliminate the pollutants that you do ingest via what you eat, drink, inhale or put on your skin. Reframe how you see the lines on your face or the stretch marks on your tummy and hips to view them in a more positive light. See the gift in them! You may also like to try an antioxidant-rich oil to nourish your skin from the inside out. Some plant oils have been shown to help boost collagen regeneration.

CYCLE CHANGES

Apply what you've learned to support the liver (refer to page 91)—fewer liver loaders going in, plenty of vegetables being consumed as well as additional liver support in the form of herbal medicine. If you are starting to overheat, taking a break from alcohol will likely prove highly beneficial. Support the adrenals (refer to page 146) by consuming less or no caffeine, exploring your perception of pressure and urgency, and embracing a breath-focused practice. Also examine your requirements for safety (refer to page 127) to help your endocrine and nervous systems to receive the message that you are safe. Additional medicinal herbs that can be highly beneficial across the peri-menopause and menopause years include rhodiola, saffron, skullcap and shatavari.

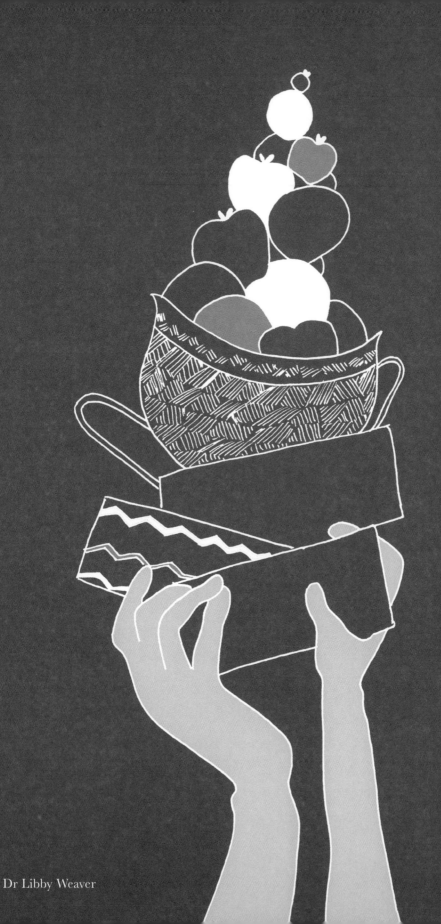

Dr Libby Weaver

WHAT CAN YOU DELEGATE?

I know when I first started to ask this question, my brain gave me an emphatic 'nothing!'. Yet when you dig a little deeper, the tasks to delegate and the people to support you *are* there. Consider that when you say you don't have time for something, what you are really staying is: that is just not a priority for me at the moment. Try it on for size and see if you are comfortable with that. The truth of this statement can help you let some things go that are less important to you, so you can embrace more of what is truly important to you. Also remember that the opposite of stress is trust (refer to page 147) and this alone helps us all to experience less tension, to relax and soften.

MUSCLE MASS

From the age of 30 onwards, you lose muscle mass unless you actively do something to prevent this. The less muscle mass we have the slower our metabolic rate. The lower your muscle mass, the less storage capacity you have for glycogen, the storage form of glucose, so the more likely you are to store excess carbohydrates as body fat. Or the more likely you are to experience blood glucose highs and lows and the sugar cravings that go with that. Prioritise building muscle mass across your whole life. This means resistance training, yoga, Pilates, carrying your luggage instead of wheeling it (as was the case up until relatively recently), carrying your groceries and children. Garden, do farm work. Use your body. Don't avoid movement.

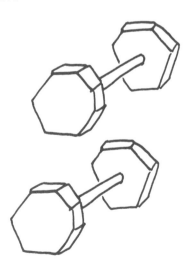

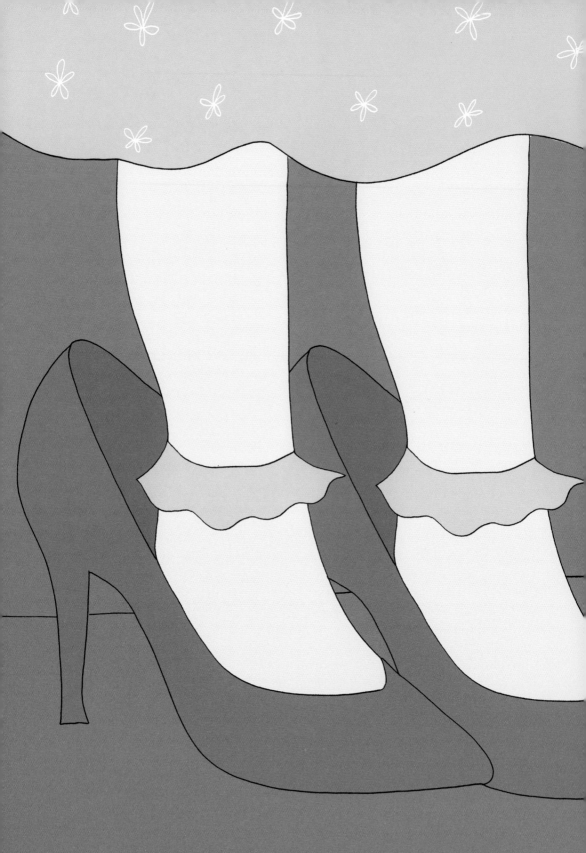

Dr Libby Weaver

Where have all the little leaders gone?

Reminding girls of their innate power

Attend any school event in New Zealand or Australia where there are children aged six, and you see many little girls who could rule the world. Their posture is upright, their eyes are bright and they have confidence in who they are—whether that is bold and boisterous or quiet and reflective. The little boys are often a bit random, shirts untucked and less mature. Hilarious and delightful of course—and I'm generalising, but you get the gist.

Return to this same school quadrangle six years later, and the difference is palpable. Strength and confidence has grown in many of the boys, while for too many girls, I cannot help but wonder where all of those little leaders have gone.

On a speaking job a few years ago, this topic came up in the green room among a group of women who want to change this pathway for girls. My curiosity about why this happens prompted questions to circle the group. Sadly, the only real answer we came up with is that little girls become aware of their bodies in ways little boys don't (if this happens for boys it happens later when some develop visible muscles and others don't). Or perhaps it is just as much about the vast difference in social acceptability that still exists between male and female sexuality. Many beliefs are born around puberty about what is okay and not okay when it comes to how we feel, what we do and ways to be.

So why is it, in this day and age, where we know so much and care so much, that this is still happening? Why do little girls feel judged by their appearance and start comparing themselves to others at such a young age? How is it possible that eight-year-olds want to go on a diet? And what can we do to minimise the self-doubt, sadness, harm and suffering for young girls?

I don't have clear answers for this. I write about this here simply to prompt more conversations about this and to foster what I hope is greater awareness of how we speak to young girls.

We need to nurture a belief in themselves within them so that they are less vulnerable to the judgements and passing comments of others.

What I do know is that our beliefs become visible on the outside in how we carry ourselves—the wrinkles we eventually get from repeated facial expressions, the way we behave and through the choices we make. Never underestimate the power of these beliefs. They form subconsciously from the repetition of external messages, the meanings we create from what people say and the expressions on their faces, as well as social conditioning. You can start to hear children's beliefs in their language patterns: 'I'm not smart', 'I'm not pretty', 'I'll never be any good at gymnastics'. And these are just the ones we hear.

The thing about beliefs is that we don't even know we've taken them on as our truth, but then they act as a filtering system for how we see, feel and experience our environment—as well as ourselves. And the brain always looks to prove itself right—we only ever see the evidence to support what we perceive and we miss all the evidence for how what we believe is not true. It's not that you consciously go around looking for opportunities to prove to yourself that you're, say, not pretty, but if you believe this about yourself you will reinforce it within every new experience.

Let's say you secretly fancy someone from work and you run into them when out one night having a drink with a friend and they pay more attention to your friend than they do to you. Rather than just thinking that attraction works in mysterious ways, you tell yourself it's because you're not as pretty as your friend. In this way, over time, our beliefs are reinforced.

By the time we are seven, psychology 101 teaches us that we have all absorbed a belief (or numerous beliefs) that we are not something enough—not good enough, not tall enough, not pretty enough, not quiet enough, not loud enough, not smart enough—just not okay the way that we are. And I can't help but dream that one day we live in a world where every child grows up (safe, well-nourished and) knowing that they are enough. For when we believe we are enough, we inherently know that we have enough. And that would change the trajectory of the future of the planet, not to mention the difference this would make among our local communities.

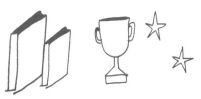

LET'S TELL OUR GIRLS THEY ARE BEAUTIFUL BUT ALSO FOCUS ON ALL THE OTHER QUALITIES THAT WE SEE IN THEM—THEIR KINDNESS, THEIR LEADERSHIP, THEIR STRENGTH.

Yet the flipside of all of this is that our voids create our values, and if it was actually possible to grow up without the 'wounds', it's unlikely that we'd ever do anything. For if you pull the veil back on so much of what we all do, it is in order to be accepted, to be liked, appreciated. To be loved. By others, or in an attempt to convince ourselves that we are worthwhile and worthy.

As I said, I don't have answers for this at the moment. I just see so much unnecessary suffering among young girls these days and it is heartbreaking. With the way our brain is at this point in human evolution, and the way we currently develop emotional maturity, it does not yet seem possible to avoid these early self-limiting beliefs, no matter whether it is chaotic or calm at home, at school, at sport and socially. So don't feel guilty—that is futile. On some level we have to trust in the journey of an individual and support them to see that, through pain, we learn and grow. And that the pain can foster an ability to contribute those learnings back to the world so that hopefully the next generation suffers less and evolves to be able to learn and contribute via other stimuli.

I'm full of hope. What I do know or certainly believe is possible is that we can encourage a strong sense of self-belief by choosing how we compliment and validate our young girls. Let's tell them that we trust in them to make excellent decisions, that we believe in them to become whatever they set their hearts to.

Let's tell them they are beautiful but also focus on all the other qualities that we see in them—their kindness, their leadership, their strength.

WE MAY NOT BE ABLE TO STOP OUR GIRLS FROM EXPERIENCING PAIN, BUT WE CAN INSTIL IN THEM A SENSE OF BELIEF THAT THEY ARE CAPABLE OF FACING AND HANDLING ANYTHING LIFE THROWS AT THEM.

For now, let's do what we can through how we communicate. Through remembering that, when we judge, it is a reflection of a perception of lack in us, not in the person we are judging, and teach children the same. To have awareness of their words and the intention behind what they express both verbal and written ('What were you hoping would be the outcome of saying/posting/writing that?'), as well as how to understand comparison and judgement. If we, as adults, raise our consciousness, it will ripple on through to the next generation and foster young girls to maintain (rather than lose and have to regain) their authentic confidence and that gentle, tender, genuine self-belief that shines in the six-year-olds in the schoolyard ∎

SKIN, hair

& NAILS

Understanding your skin

Appreciate its abilities

___

EPIDERMIS:

The outermost layer of skin is brand new every 28 to 35 days. The older we get, the longer it tends to take to replace the outside layer. The epidermis is made of dead skin cells that were born at the bottom of the second layer of skin, called the dermis. Sebum forms the acid mantle on the surface of the epidermis, a film to help protect bacteria and viruses from penetrating the surface and getting down into the pores. You want the skin to work as the magnificent organ it is, rather than disrupt it, so a first great step to supporting better skin is not damaging the acid mantle with what you use to wash your face. You'll come to learn more about this in later chapters.

Two to three per cent of the cells that make up the epidermis are melanocytes (1), the cells that provide pigment to the skin. Some people notice that irregularities in skin colour start to appear if the epidermis is treated with harsh peels or synthetic chemicals. This is due to the deformation of the melanocytes (1). Again, we want to care for, nourish and support our skin, not punish it. And I hope this book helps you to do this.

DERMIS:

Brand new baby skin cells are born at the bottom of this layer of the skin. The best way to imagine the life of a skin cell is this: when they are born, they pick up information from their local environment. For example, are there all nutrients available, or are some missing?

Historically, a major reason a nutrient would be missing is because of a famine. Your new baby skin cell doesn't know that you might be missing some key nutrients because you eat in a restricted way, or live on too many processed foods and takeaways. It thinks there is a famine. Likewise if the skin cell picks up on hormonal information present, such as stress hormones. If there are more stress hormones than love hormones present, then they think your life is in danger, as stress hormones have always communicated threat to the body. As these brand new skin cells begin their 28 to 35 days' migration to the outside of the body, they transform into what are known as keratinocytes. Once they reach the outside of the body and are exposed to oxygen they die. So when we approach skin appearance from the outside in, you are trying to work on dead skin cells!

Of course there are products now that can penetrate that outside layer, but you get the gist. Often what we try to change from the outside in would actually respond to a beauty from the inside out approach, which was why I wrote a book of that name. Your insides create your outside.

Keratinocytes produce protein so that whenever the skin is cut or grazed, healing can happen efficiently. They also send signals to the dermis to start producing more new cells to help with this so the skin can knit back together (1). Isn't that clever? The dermis can also be thought of as 'water world', as this layer helps to keep tissues hydrated, vital to clear, glowing skin.

SUBCUTANEOUS TISSUE:

This layer houses blood vessels, fatty tissue and muscle tissue which all perform critical tasks in maintaining healthy skin. The muscle and fat act as shock absorbers for the skin, in a similar way to collagen, as you will see over the page where we look at how a wrinkle forms. This is also the layer where we might find bands of cellulite, which is essentially fat, often housing old problematic substances that we've eaten (think pesticides) or produced ourselves (think estrogen) that the body couldn't get rid of efficiently. It s held in place by connective tissue lined with fat.

THE OUTERMOST LAYER OF SKIN IS BRAND NEW EVERY 28 TO 35 DAYS. THE OLDER WE GET, THE LONGER IT TENDS TO TAKE TO REPLACE THE OUTSIDE LAYER.

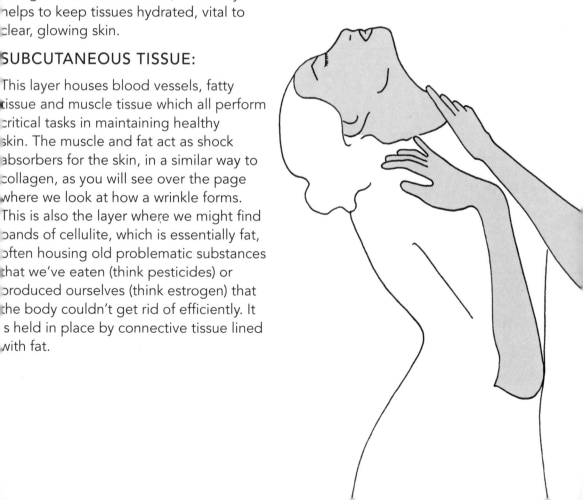

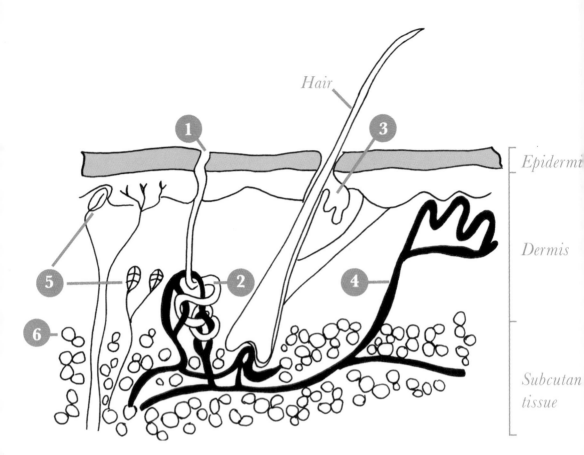

Hair

1

3

Epidermi

Dermis

5

2

4

6

Subcutan
tissue

1 PORE

There are a number of different types of pores. Some deliver sweat to the surface of the skin, while others transport sebum. They can deliver scent as well. In this illustration, it is sweat being transported. Think of pores as openings for important fluids to reach the surface of the body. Problems only occur with pores if they are infiltrated by too many bacteria (usually feeding on sebum), not due to sweat or sebum themselves, although there are hormonal scenarios when sebum production can become excessive—at puberty, for example. The fluids travelling up towards the pore can also carry dead skin cells with them. This can add to the accumulation of sebum, giving the bacteria more to feed on and leading to potential problems, such as acne.

2 SWEAT GLAND

These play a major role in supporting the body to regulate temperature, by providing perspiration to be transported to the surface of the body. As sweat dries it helps to cool the body.

Sweat is mostly water; however, it contains mineral salts that can leave a salty crust on the skin once the water has evaporated. It travels in a duct to the surface of the skin and is released via a pore. It can also carry problematic substances out of the body, which is a wonderful help!

3 SEBACEOUS GLAND

These glands produce sebum, the substance that keeps skin nourished, lubricated and moist (as opposed to dry). It is made of fatty acids, fatty alcohols, waxes, lactic acid and salts and has a pH of between 4.3 and 6, meaning it is slightly acidic and it needs to be (1). The sebum helps form the protective layer on the outside of the epidermis known as the 'acid mantle', whose job it is to neutralise bacteria so they can't penetrate into the pores, causing congestion. Sebum travels to the surface of the body along the hair shaft and an open, functioning pore allows the sebum to reach the outside of the skin (the epidermis) to do its critical work of sealing moisture into the skin. We would dry out without sebum! So if you ever feel frustrated by body hair in certain places, you could flip it in your mind and instead feel grateful that sebum has a way to reach the surface of your skin!

5 NERVE ENDING

These allow us to feel! Imagine if you didn't have the sense of touch. Be sure to appreciate the senses you have every day! They bring such joy and so many experiences to our lives. Nerve endings also act as sensors for heat and cold, letting us know when to put on or take off layers of clothing or when to start sweating. They also help protect us from extreme, harsh temperatures—think fire or snow.

4 BLOOD CAPILLARY

One of the main jobs of the capillaries is to deliver oxygen and nutrients to the skin. What a vital task! You want highly nourished blood, to which eating whole, real foods enormously contributes. Iron, in particular, is needed for the transport of oxygen throughout the body, including delivery of it in the blood capillaries supporting the skin. You also want healthy blood vessels in general, which means minimising how much sugar you eat, as elevated blood glucose levels can damage the lining of the vessels. In time, this can impact the appearance and health of the skin.

6 FATTY TISSUE

There is supposed to be fat here. There is also muscle tissue to support skin structure. However, from the age of 30 onwards, muscle mass from anywhere in the body, including the skin support muscles, starts to decline. This allows the infiltration of more fat, and often fat that is used as a storage house for problematic substances that the body couldn't fully detoxify so they could leave the body. The loss of muscle and the increase in fatty tissue can also occur more hastily if/when we produce excessive amounts of a chronic stress hormone: cortisol. The health and appearance of the skin really is influenced by so much else going on inside the body!

How does a wrinkle form?

———

Traversing the dermis are fibrous strands, about 80 per cent of which are made of a protein called collagen (1). It forms a dense matrix (that you can see in illustration 1) that protects the skin from splitting when it is stretched. The remainder of the strands are elastin, another protein-based fibre. It acts like rubber bands (1) so that whenever the skin is pulled, elastin draws it back into its original shape. As we age, the elastin tends to weaken. Collagen and elastin are supposed to be moist and plump, which makes the skin appear full, soft and unlined—typically how it appears when we are young.

These fibres give skin its fullness and shape and as we age, they can be damaged by free radicals. This leads them to shrink and cross-link with other collagen strands, forming structures that, if you could see them, look like fish netting. As the collagen base shrinks,

the skin at the surface folds over itself forming wrinkles (1), as you can see in illustration 3. If this process continues unhindered, the skin itself can look like fish netting, if the collagen becomes excessively cross-linked.

Remember that the antidote to the challenge of free radicals is the antioxidants found predominantly in coloured plant foods, so be sure to amp up your consumption of those masterful, protective and nourishing substances.

Vitamin C is of particular importance to both maintaining collagen, preventing its breakdown, as well as in building new collagen. Good food sources of vitamin C include citrus fruits, kiwifruit, capsicum or you might like to add a food-based vitamin C supplement.

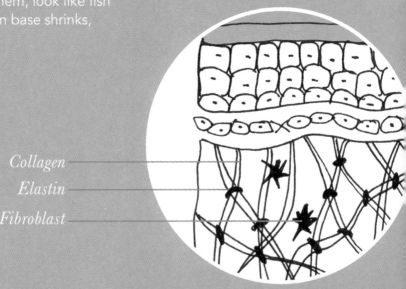

Collagen —————

Elastin —————

Fibroblast —————

1

You can see that the surface of the skin is smooth and flat and that there is a high density of collagen and elastin below the surface supporting the top layer. You will also notice plenty of fibroblasts, cells that produce collagen and other fibres. The more of these present, the better your ability to regenerate new collagen, provided you have adequate vitamin C available.

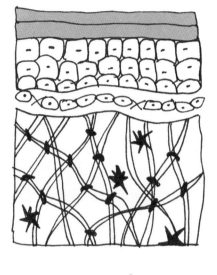

2

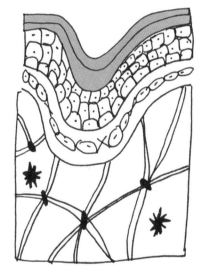

The skin is starting to fold in on itself due to the collagen and elastin starting to degrade. There are also fewer fibroblasts, meaning there is now a decreased ability to regenerate new structural fibres to support the appearance of the skin.

3

A wrinkle has now formed and there is a lack of collagen and elastin. There are even fewer fibroblasts at this stage in wrinkle formation.

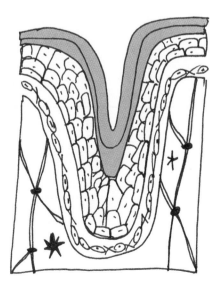

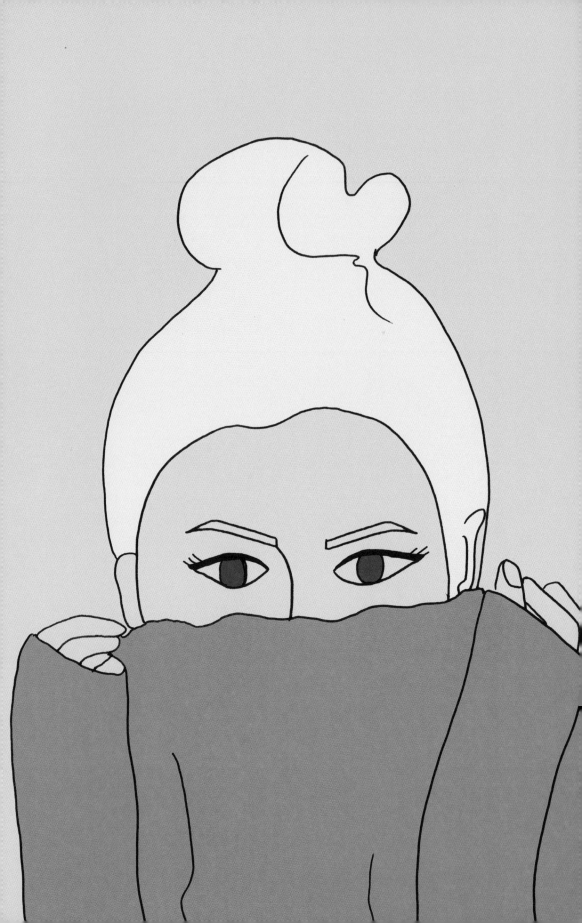

Are you aggravated by acne?

How to resolve it for good

Acne involves much more than just the skin—it involves numerous body systems. It can bring much heartache and frustration to someone experiencing it, so let's understand it and piece together the steps to take that will help resolve and heal it. It is important to first understand the actual processes that create acne, for then you can see why I suggest what I do to help your skin's condition.

Acne occurs when the sebaceous glands become overactive and a collection of sebum blocks hair follicles and pores. As you learnt earlier, the newly born skin cells, most of which are keratinocytes, migrate outward from the lower levels of the skin (refer to page 52). If the hair follicles and pores are blocked with sebum, the new cells trying to make their way to the surface get bogged.

These cells don't live for very long, so soon they die, and they become trapped in the follicles and pores. The excess sebum and dead cells form a plug, or a blackhead, in the pore, which prevents the usual drainage of the oil (1). The accumulation of excess sebum gives the bacteria of the skin more to feed on, so they too multiply and hence large populations gather and feed on

the sebum. This irritates the skin and eventually tends to cause infections, which is how a pimple or pustule occurs (1). The bacterial species most commonly linked to acne is *Propionibacterium acnes*.

Other factors are involved in this cycle as well. Sex hormone imbalances, particularly a surge in androgen levels (male sex hormones that occur in boys and girls for the first time at puberty) increase the production of sebum, which tends to mean more blocked pores and infections and, in turn, creates pustules— and the acne cycle continues until a step in this process is disrupted. Usually this means addressing sex hormones (due to their triggering of excess sebum production) via improving digestive system function, dietary changes, correcting nutritional deficiencies, as well as hormone clearance from the body, which is the job of the liver.

Poor digestion adds a load to the liver and kidneys. When digestion isn't functioning optimally, the liver and kidneys aren't able to filter the higher levels of hormones in the blood efficiently. These processes must improve to prevent the hormones stimulating additional sebum production. I have seen countless cases of acne improve and then resolve with a commitment to caring for and supporting the digestive system, liver and kidneys. Zinc supplementation is almost always necessary, not only for its role in sex hormone regulation, but also for immune function and its wound-healing/scar-reduction capabilities.

Emotionally, acne can be very challenging. Most people with acne will say to me that they dislike themselves. They have expanded the dislike that would have initially been for the pustules to themselves as individuals. I work to help them see that their deep sadness or immense frustration with themselves (their skin) can become a gift, for it is almost always our body trying to wake us up to eat, drink, move, think, breathe, believe, or perceive differently.

And learning whatever this is really about can literally change the course of your life! From an emotional perspective, and the third pillar of my work, given that acne typically appears during adolescence, I can't help but wonder if it is in some way linked to feeling socially insecure or feeling lousy about yourself and having a harsh inner voice that criticises because you feel like you always let yourself down (which may indicate that it would be highly beneficial for you to examine your expectations).

The self-deprecation ideally needs to transform into appreciation.

TOO MANY PRECIOUS PEOPLE HAVE FORGOTTEN THAT THEY ARE PRECIOUS.

They can no longer see their own beauty, caught up instead in their perceived flaws. I find, if the person can accept where they are (and I know that is a big ask) and begin to work with what is—and if they start eating in a way that serves them as an individual (though I share some common solutions that may help on the next page), along with taking some herba medicine liver support—improvements in the skin begin. And this is so encouraging for the person that they are usually happy to continue with their new routine of self-nurturing and self-care.

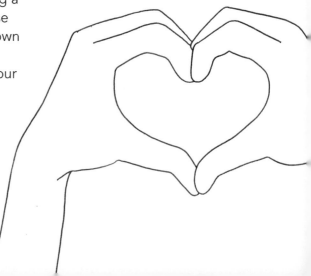

Dr Libby Weaver

STEPS TO RESOLVE ACNE

Eat whole real foods only. Cut the refined sugar and anything artificial: sweeteners, flavours, colours, preservatives.

Don't disrupt the acid mantle of your skin with how you wash your skin. Your skin is not supposed to be 'squeaky clean' after you cleanse it. Squeaky clean feels tight, and for oily skin, this results in the skin producing even more oil (sebum) to compensate. You don't want to send the skin this signal. The acid mantle is your skin's protection against bacteria and when it is disrupted, they can enter the pores and keep the cycle going. Nourish and nurture your skin back to health with non-synthetic products that support its function, rather than those that interfere with this. Refer to page 235 for more about skincare.

Make water your main drink. No soft drinks at all.

Take liver herbs to support the efficient clearance of sex hormones from the body.

Take a food-based zinc supplement.

• Many people with acne need a strict dairy-free diet for a minimum of three months to break the cycle. When you trial the reintroduction of dairy products after this period, if the skin worsens (is noticeably redder or more pustules form again, after a period of improvement), the period without it needs to extend. See an experienced nutrition professional if this is the case to ensure all of your nutrient needs are being met.

• If you don't get your periods regularly, herbal medicine can help the pituitary communicate more effectively with the ovaries. Combining the herbs paeonia and licorice (the herb not the lolly!) or chaste tree (vitex), can be helpful. It can be wise to work with a nutritionist or medical herbalist to assist you in establishing a regular cycle. Stress management is almost always needed for this too (refer to page 146).

• If you feel that there is an emotional component to your acne, you might find it helpful to speak to a wise, trusted friend, sibling or parent, a counsellor or psychologist to help bring you a new perspective to a situation or how you see yourself.

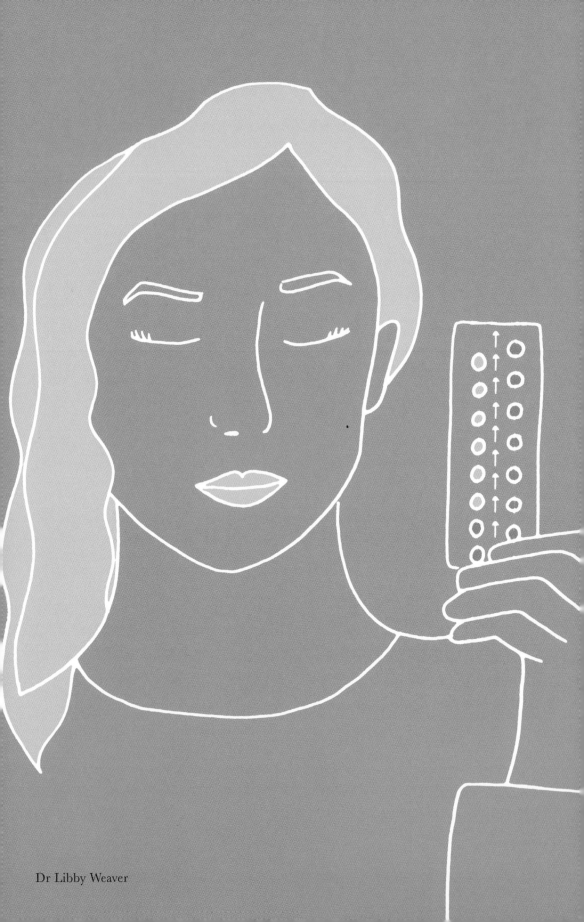

Dr Libby Weaver

Is the pill the only thing between you and a breakout?

How to break this cycle

Some teenagers and young women are prescribed the oral contraceptive pill (OCP), not for contraception or even to help with painful periods, but to manage their skin. As a result, as adult women, they often worry what will happen to their skin if they come off the pill. Let's explore what's involved in this scenario.

Please let me begin by saying that I am not anti-medication. There are times when the pill is the right decision for someone. What concerns me is when it is used to mask something else that is occurring, solely because the mechanisms that created the problem (the skin challenge) in the first place won't have been corrected. And this not only matters in the short term, but very much in the long term.

There is no doubt that sex hormones can have a significant impact on the skin. It might be puberty when you first noticed your skin became congested or unpredictable, or perhaps it breaks out a few days (or a week) before you menstruate. Or maybe the breakouts started around puberty and they've never really gone away. Or perhaps your skin cleared up after some challenging changes in the teenage years, only to perplexingly return in adult life years or decades later. Very rarely is the problem with the ovaries themselves. Usually the problem lies with the signals the ovaries are on the receiving end of (from the pituitary gland and other endocrine glands), and/or the mechanisms involved in the clearance of sex hormones from the body (liver and bowels).

The job of the OCP is to prevent ovulation and it does this by supplying the body with post-ovulation levels of synthetic estrogen and a synthetic form of progesterone. Hormones from the pituitary gland govern ovulation when a woman is not on the pill. However, because the levels of sex hormones from the OCP in the blood constantly communicate to the pituitary that ovulation has taken place, it does not surge luteinising hormone (LH) or follicle stimulating hormone (FSH), which are required for ovulation. In simple terms, the pituitary ceases to communicate to the ovaries and the ovaries, as a result, don't do much at all since ovulation is suppressed.

But if your skin breaks out (without the pill), the body is letting you know that something is awry. It could be that something isn't quite right with your innate levels of estrogen, progesterone, LH, FSH, testosterone (or other androgens) and/or your body's current ability to convert cholesterol into its end products, which include estrogen, progesterone, testosterone and cortisol (refer to the flowchart that shows these biochemical pathways). And the pill doesn't correct this. It shuts down the communication between the pituitary and the ovaries.

Years or decades later, you decide you want to come off the pill to take a break or because you want to conceive. For some women, it can take only a few months for the communication pathways to be re-established, while for others it takes years. It seems for others still, that pituitary ovarian communication remains disrupted long term. This scenario can contribute to immense sadness or frustration for a couple wanting to conceive. I have sadly seen this time and time again.

Conception aside, what if you simply want to take a break from the OCP, but you're worried about your skin breaking out? That was why you went on the pill in the first place, after all. Or perhaps you've had breaks before and, every time you give it a go, your skin breaks out again. My suggestion is you do some work on

the systems that support good hormonal balance for at least three months before you come off the pill.

For these three months, you can't restore your own innate levels of estrogen, progesterone, LH or FSH because the pill will keep all of those low. What you can do is support the liver and the adrenals. Adrenal support is necessary because it is the only place you make real progesterone from while you are on the OCP. This is because the pill prevents ovulation and the main place you make your own progesterone from is the crater (called the corpus luteum) that remains on the surface of the ovary after you ovulate in the second half of your cycle. And you need the liver support to clear problematic substances (refer to page 88 for more on this), as well as the synthetic estrogen from the body, via the urine and faeces. This is so they aren't recycled and either drive inflammation or become stored in body fat.

Adrenal support varies in its focus in this behind-the-scenes restoration process, however, a great first step is to decrease stress hormone production. 'Easier said than done!' you exclaim. Refer to the strategies outlined on page 146 to help get you started. Useful medicinal herbs include Siberian ginseng, withania, licorice, and skullcap (for its anti-anxiety actions).

For liver support, refer to the ideas on page 91. Useful medicinal herbs include

t Mary's thistle, globe artichoke, broccoli
prouts and bupleurum. Having worked
vith people for 20 years, I have also
bserved that a strict dairy-free trial
hot permanently, unless a nutrition
professional warrants this necessary for
ou) for the three-month 'preparing to
ome off the pill' time, as well as for the
rst two months without it, can really help
eep the skin calm. I am yet to decipher
he mechanism behind this—I have a
umber of theories, but they are just that
t the moment. I just know what I've seen
hake an enormous difference in clinical
ractice. To be without dairy foods for
hore than three months, it is wise to
ee a nutritional professional to ensure
ll your nutrient needs are being met
om the other foods you are choosing.
upplementation of essential fatty acids
EFAs) can also be helpful as they help to
hitigate inflammation.

cannot encourage you enough to persist
your desire for and pursuit of clear skin,
ot only for the confidence that tends to
ring people, but for the inner health and
armony it reflects.

This flow chart shows how some
cholesterol in the body is converted
into progesterone. Many factors then
contribute to the decision about
how much progesterone to hold as
progesterone and how much to convert
into testosterone, a form of estrogen
(estrone or estradiol) and/or cortisol.
Please note, there are numerous
intermediary steps in these pathways,
but for ease of understanding they have
been omitted.

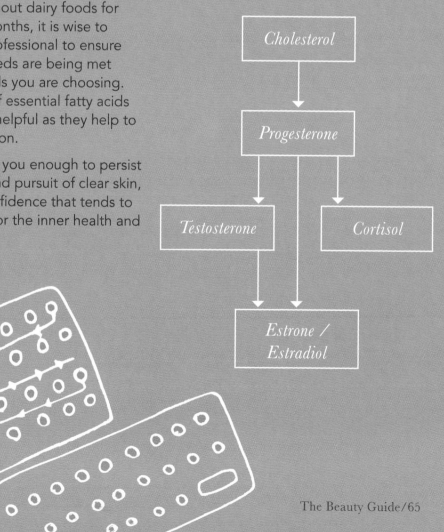

How to get the glow

The natural way to radiant skin

—

When you see someone (in real life, not via filters!) with a glowing complexion, it springs from much deeper within them than some type of clever highlighter they've applied or the primer they put on that morning. Skin that truly glows is cultivated from a vast array of physical and emotional processes inside you, including the nutrients you supply your body with as well as how lit up you feel about your life. Everything, even what you are focused on in this very moment, tends to be reflected on the outside and contributes (or not) to your sparkle. Here are some tips on how you can get that true radiant glow shining from deep within.

1 Change your pillowcase regularly.

2 Try an oil-based product, rich in topical antioxidants, to moisturise and help protect your skin. Press it in with your fingertips rather than rubbing it in.

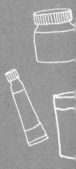

3 If you wear makeup, remove it before bed. Always.

4 Don't use substances on your skin that disrupt the skin's natural acid mantle. When you think about skincare, think of nourishing your skin, not punishing your skin. Gentle, not harsh.

5 Make water your main drink and be sure to drink enough each day to stay hydrated; your thirst is your guide. The dermis stores the water for your skin, keeping it hydrated and plump. Your urine is your blood having been filtered by your kidneys, and it is yet another mechanism through which waste products leave your body.

6 Don't add to the synthetic chemical load of your body via what you put on your skin. Refer to page 235 for more on this.

7 The skin particularly loves vitamin C—found in citrus fruits, kiwifruit, capsicum, and raw brassica vegies. You might like to add a food-based supplement to boost your intake.

8 If you have a specific skin complaint, use the strategies suggested in the skin section of the Beauty Solutions chapter, beginning on page 208.

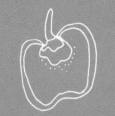

9 Quit sugar. In other words, omit processed foods and drinks and only eat whole, real foods, including plenty of plants. Trial it for 4 weeks and notice how it enhances your glow!

10 The skin loves it when your bowels and liver are working optimally (explained on page 93). If you don't use your bowels daily, make this your number-one priority and consider adding extra liver support via medicinal herbs such as St Mary's thistle, globe artichoke and turmeric.

11 On waking, place your hands on your heart and connect to the gift of life—what a blessing it is that you get another day!

12 Don't touch your face unless you've washed your hands!

13 If you experience skin congestion, pimples, cysts under the skin, or rosacea, for example, do a dairy-free diet trial for 4 weeks to see if that begins to make difference. That means omitting all dairy products, not just milk. If it makes no ifference, the dairy can come back. If your skin improves or clears up and you want to ontinue with this new way of eating, consult an experienced nutrition professional to nsure you are obtaining all the nutrients you need to stay healthy and full of energy.

14 Eat plenty of antioxidant-rich plants. icture a platter filled with oods of the colours of the ainbow. That platter packs a assive antioxidant punch!

15 Consider taking an additional food-based, antioxidant-rich organic greens powder, and/or supplemental essential fatty acids, particularly DHA.

16 Less stress, more trust (in the unfolding of life). Refer to page 146 for more on this.

17 Let yourself have what you already have—the night sky, for xample. It's what joy is all about, and y allows us to see and experience even ore beauty within ourselves and the orld.

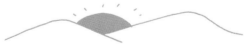

18 Ask yourself: 'What lights me up?' and work out how you bring more of that into your daily life.

19 ust before bed, ank yourself r your day.

20 Be You!

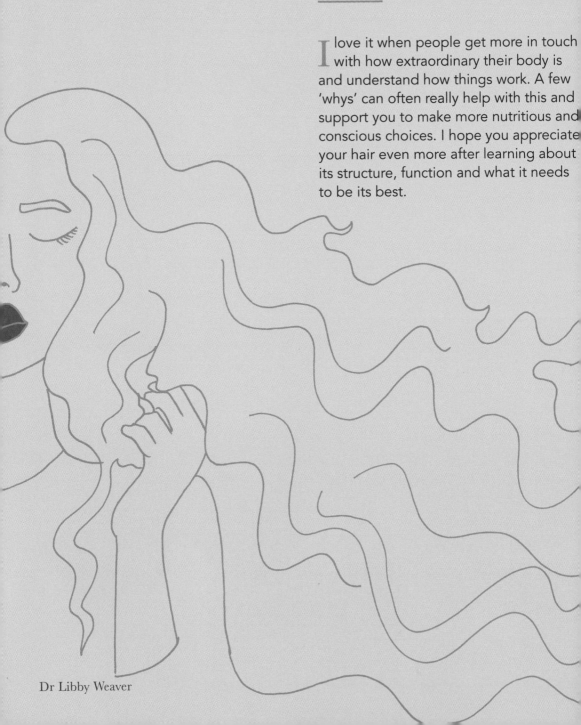

Luscious locks

Understanding your hair

———

I love it when people get more in touch with how extraordinary their body is and understand how things work. A few 'whys' can often really help with this and support you to make more nutritious and conscious choices. I hope you appreciate your hair even more after learning about its structure, function and what it needs to be its best.

Dr Libby Weaver

Human hair is made of keratin, which is made from amino acids, and dead skin cells. Its primary function is to prevent heat loss from a person's head; plus, it transfers sensory information. It also acts as an excretory mechanism for the body.

At the time I was doing my PhD, which examined nutritional and biochemical factors in children with autism spectrum disorder (ASD), a study was published by another research group. It assessed the heavy metal content of hair from children before the age of five, comparing those who went on to develop ASD to those who didn't develop any conditions. Initially, a potential conclusion from the study could be that heavy metals were not involved in the aetiology of ASD as the researchers found that the children with ASD had significantly lower levels of heavy metals in their hair compared to the control group (1). However, after additional research, the scientists released a statement about what their research meant.

They said that children without ASD had higher levels of heavy metals in their hair because they were able to excrete them from the body more efficiently than children with ASD, and that children with ASD potentially had higher levels of heavy metals stored in their body and were unable to use the hair as a mechanism of excretion as effectively as children without ASD (2). This research was a great reminder to me that the body works to excrete the substances it doesn't require or those that may be toxic at high levels. Hair is yet another way the body does this.

HAIR STRUCTURE AND GROWTH

Hair is made up of two separate structures: the follicle in the skin and the shaft that we can see. Refer to the picture that shows how the hair grows out of the skin on page 54. The follicle is a stocking-like structure that contains several layers with different roles. A projection forms at the base of each follicle and, if you could see it, it looks like a finger being pushed a small distance through the bottom of a stocking (3). This stalk is called a papilla and it contains tiny blood vessels that feed the cells. The bulb, which is the bottom part surrounding the papilla, is alive and it is the only part fed by the capillaries (3), the efficiency of which can be interfered with by stress hormones, as you will come to know on page 103. The cells in the bulb divide every 24 to 72 hours, which is particularly rapid.

An inner and outer sheath surround the follicle, whose job it is to both shape and protect the growing hair shaft. The inner sheath follows the hair shaft and ends below the opening of a sebaceous gland (which produces the oily secretion known as sebum) and sometimes a sweat gland (3). A muscle is attached to the outer sheath and when this muscle contracts, it drives the hair to stand up. You'll notice this sensation when you experience goosebumps.

As you already understand, sebum is incredibly important for the skin and the same is true for the hair as it acts like a natural conditioner. We make differing amounts of sebum across our life stages. For example, more sebum starts to be produced as puberty begins, while many adult women describe a turning point, at varying ages or after very challenging times, when they notice sebum production starts to decrease.

Also think about what might happen when we kill hair follicles, either on purpose or accidentally. Females tend to like lustrous locks on their head but not in many (if any) other places. A variety of modalities are used these days to get rid of hair—temporarily like waxing or more permanently like laser treatments. Yet sebum is delivered to the exterior of the skin via hairs, so if enough follicles are permanently damaged, what happens to the conditioning of the skin? Is it just reduced or destroyed in that area? We don't yet really fully understand the long-term consequences of permanent hair removal as it is still too new.

HAIR ON THE SCALP GROWS ABOUT 15 CENTIMETRES PER YEAR, WHICH EQUATES TO ABOUT 0.3 TO 0.4 MILLIMETRES PER DAY.

Human hair loss and growth is random and not seasonal or cyclic, unlike other mammals. A random number of hairs will be in various stages of shedding and growth, the latter stages of which are known as catagen, telogen and anagen.

1. THE CATAGEN (TRANSITION THAT SIGNIFIES THE END OF THE HAIR GROWTH) PHASE:

Three per cent of all hairs are in this phase at any time. The duration of this phase is about two to three weeks.

2. THE TELOGEN (SHEDDING) PHASE:

Ten to 15 per cent of all hairs are typically in this stage at any given time. This phase lasts for about 100 days for hairs on the scalp. This phase lasts much longer for eyebrow, eyelash, arm and leg hair. About 25 to 100 telogen hairs are typically shed each day.

3. THE ANAGEN (HAIR GROWTH) PHASE:

The cells in the root of the hair divide rapidly at this stage. During this phase the hair grows about one centimetre every 28 days. Scalp hair stays in this active phase of growth for two to six years.

If you have difficulty growing your hair beyond a certain length, it can be due to a short active phase of growth, while people whose hair seems to grow quickly and easily tend to have a longer active phase of growth. Eyebrow, eyelash, arm and leg hairs have a growth phase of about 30 to 45 days, which is quite short; this is the main reason why these hairs are so much shorter than scalp hair.

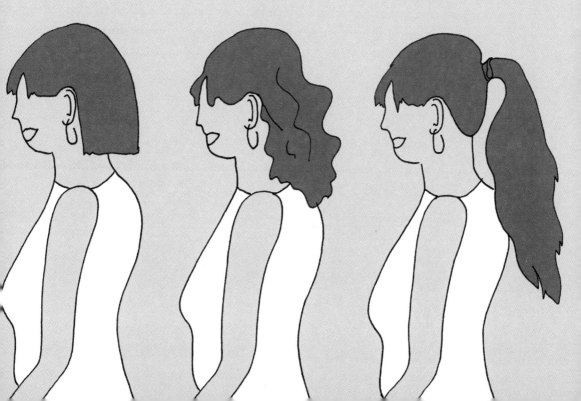

HEALTHY HAIR

Like all the other aspects of beauty, healthy hair is first dependent on great digestion, particularly protein digestion. Good protein digestion relies on good stomach acid production and for this you need to chew your food well, eat in a calm state and ideally not consume caffeine or water 30 minutes before or after eating. You can also stimulate stomach acid production by consuming apple cider vinegar or lemon juice in warm water 5–20 minutes before eating.

I have also found that when undesirable changes to the hair are occurring, the adrenals usually need support. This is explained in the section about stress, as well as on page 83, which explores more Eastern philosophies of lustrous hair.

HAIR NUTRITION

All—yes all—nutrients contribute in some way to the health of the hair. Some specific examples include:

Split ends are the result of the dead cells that make the hair flake apart. Vitamin C has been shown to slow down the formation of split ends and help hair that breaks easily.

Mechanical, chemical and heat stress (blow drying and hair straighteners) can also lead to split ends, so it's important to consume the nutrients that help to keep the hair nourished and prevent dryness such as the essential fatty acids (EFAs). Your hair will love them.

If hair becomes finer over time, this can be due to shrinkage of the hair follicles. Vitamin D plays a critical role in hair follicle maintenance and healing.

If the hair becomes oily out of the blue, sex hormone balance usually needs to be addressed, which often involves support for the adrenals and liver (refer to pages 146 and 91 respectively for more information about this), plus I discuss this is detail in my book *Women's Wellness Wisdom*.

If the hair becomes dry out of the blue, more EFAs are usually needed in the diet. If this does not rectify the dryness in about six weeks, it is worthwhile investigating thyroid function and/or iron deficiency.

Other nutrients that are essential to great hair include iron, zinc, calcium, magnesium, biotin and silica. Food sources of these nutrients are listed below (4,5).

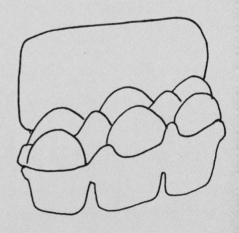

IRON

Food sources of iron include:

- red meat
- offal meat
- eggs
- legumes
- green leafy vegetables.

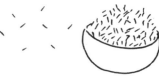

ZINC

Food sources of zinc include:

- oysters
- pumpkin seeds (pepitas)
- sunflower seeds
- red meat
- offal meat
- lentils
- eggs.

CALCIUM

Food sources of calcium include:

- sesame seeds
- salmon with edible bones
- sardines
- almonds
- green leafy vegetables
- tahini (sesame seed paste).

SILICA

Food sources of silica include:

- whole grains such as rice and oats
- fruits
- vegetables
- legumes.

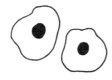

MAGNESIUM

Food sources of magnesium include:

- nuts, particularly Brazil nuts, almonds and cashews
- cacao
- seeds, particularly pumpkin seeds
- green leafy vegetables.

BIOTIN

Food sources of biotin include:

- nuts, particularly almonds and hazelnuts
- small amounts widely spread in meats and vegetables
- liver
- peanuts
- eggs
- lentils.

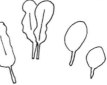
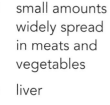
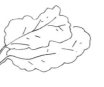

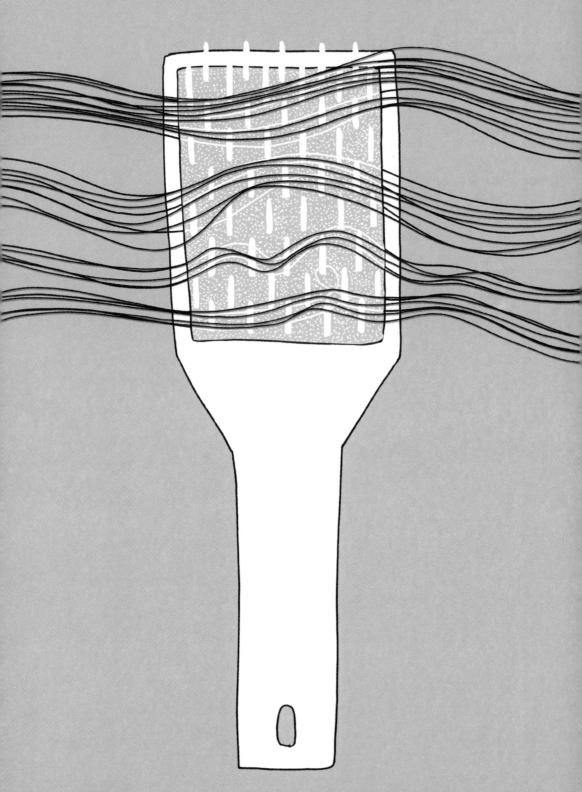

Dr Libby Weaver

Hair help

When your hair seems to be thinning

A certain amount of hair loss is to be expected as part of the natural life cycle of hair growth, but do you ever feel like you're losing what looks to be handfuls at a time? It is becoming more and more common for women to notice significant hair loss at some stage in their lives.

For some, this is just a temporary occurrence, maybe for just a few months, and usually following a period of major stress or change. Yet for others, major hair loss is continuous.

If you are losing more hair than what is considered to be a normal part of the hair cycle, you will begin to notice that your part is widening. There will also be hair on your pillow when you wake up most, if not all, mornings.

The most common causes associated with this kind of significant female hair loss include:

- iron deficiency
- poor thyroid function or thyroid disease
- polycystic ovarian syndrome (PCOS)
- hormonal contraception or replacement therapy
- after childbirth
- autoimmune alopecia
- chronic illness.

However, let's say you get tested to check all of these things and there is no confirmed cause for your hair loss. It can leave you scratching your head (pardon the pun) wondering how to resolve it. Perhaps you write it off as genetic because there's no other explanation that has presented itself. And sure, genetic predisposition can of course play a role in any health condition. However, epigenetics has taught us that the environment, namely our lifestyle choices (including the way we eat), influences whether a gene expresses itself or not.

So what are some of the other factors in the modern world that might be contributing to hair loss and that may get missed with traditional testing? In over two decades of working with women, the most common cause of hair loss in women I found, that was not a disease, was due to sex hormones. At times it was the result of some hormonal-based contraception and at others the result of changes to the sex hormone ratio (this was usually coupled with other cycle change indicators). And stress had almost always contributed to the alteration in sex hormone balance.

What the hormonally based contraception cases tended to have in common was a synthetic form of progesterone, of which there are numerous types that can behave like testosterone in the body to varying degrees.

Some types of progestins are referred to as 'androgenic' (testosterone is an androgen) and they have been shown to shrink hair follicles. It can take a long time, years even, for hair loss stemming from these synthetic hormones to become noticeable.

Chronic inflammation, as diagnosed by the elevation of markers in the blood— often generated by lifestyle factors such as a poor-quality diet, smoking and/ or chronic stress—was another feature of significant female hair loss that I observed in practice over the years. Hair improvements became evident after about three to six months of dietary change, nutritional supplementation and herbal medicine to lower the inflammatory markers.

If the basis of hair loss was associated with naturally elevated androgens (i.e. not the result of taking a contraceptive), stress-management techniques (such as incorporating regular restorative practices) and liver and adrenal support were usually needed.

If you are noticing or concerned about significant hair loss, it's important to first see your GP and rule out the medical conditions listed above.

Following are some general tips to support the regrowth of healthy hair when much has been lost. Some of these tips are also valuable to ensure you maintain excellent hair condition whether you're experiencing hair loss or not. Keep in mind that your hair tends to be a reflection of your health three to six months ago so be patient as it can take some time to improve.

Ensure you are eating in a way that is right for you. Refer to my book *What am I Supposed to Eat?* if you need help with this, or if you are confused about food, which is common these days. Considerations might include whether you digest dairy or gluten well, how much caffeine, alcohol and processed food you consume and whether you eat plenty of vegetables each day, at numerous meals.

IN OVER TWO DECADES OF WORKING WITH WOMEN, THE MOST COMMON CAUSE OF HAIR LOSS I'VE FOUND, THAT WAS NOT A DISEASE, WAS DUE TO SEX HORMONES.

Eat in a way that focuses on real food. Avoid refined sugars and starches, preservatives, sweeteners, artificial colours and deep-fried foods. Eating in a way that is rich in plant foods goes a long way to giving you the nutrients you need for great hair health. Not to mention that the substances unique to each plant support liver detoxification, immune function and help to decrease inflammation.

Promote good digestion and a healthy gut bacteria profile. Every other body system relies on the optimal functioning of the gut and your gut bacteria can create or lower inflammation.

Focus on balancing your sex hormones so that estrogen and progesterone are both high when they are supposed to be, which indicates a regular ovulation and menstrual cycle. If this is a key issue for you, learn more about how to better support adrenal and liver function, as well as ways to foster good communication between the pituitary gland and the ovaries. Refer to the section about feeling safe on page 122 for more on this.

Consider getting your zinc and iron levels ('iron studies') tested by your GP. If they are low, they must be replenished with diet and/or nutritional supplements. Zinc and iron are both needed for healthy hair follicles and they are the two most common nutritional deficiencies in the world, particularly among women of menstruation age. Food sources of zinc include oysters (very high level), red meat (moderate amount) and seeds (lower level).

Food sources of iron include red meat (highly bioavailable iron), eggs and lentils (moderate), and green vegies (lower levels).

Consult with your GP or medical specialist about exploring the use of non-hormonal methods of contraception ▪

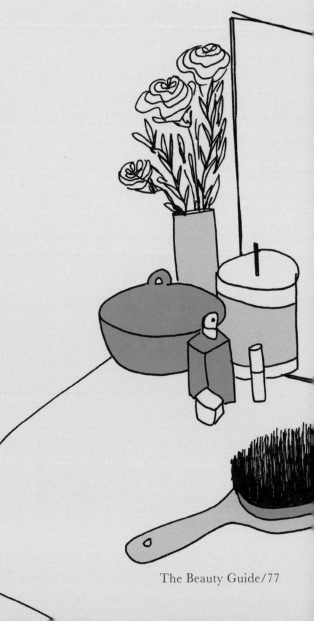

Nailing it

What your nails say about your health

____

Have you ever paused to contemplate why you have fingernails? What purpose do they serve? And have you ever wondered why they might change in appearance, strength, markings and smoothness?

Well, nails—both those of the fingers and toes—act as protective plates. Your fingernails also act to enhance the sensations of the fingertip. Each fingertip has an astronomical number of nerve endings in it, which allows us to receive volumes of information about objects we touch.

____

NAILS ACT AS A COUNTERFORCE TO THE FINGERTIP, PROVIDING EVEN MORE SENSORY INPUT WHEN WE TOUCH SOMETHING [1].

____

Nourishment is the key to creating strong healthy nails. Fingernails and toenails are made of keratin (1), a protein which is made up of amino acids. They also have minerals built into their matrix, including calcium, magnesium, zinc and boron. Good-quality dietary protein consumption is essential to nail quality and very soft nails can be the result of inadequate protein intake or poor protein utilisation by the body. The latter is typically due to poor digestion, often resulting from insufficient stomach acid production or stomach acid that is not low enough in its pH.

Alterations in the appearance of nails can be a reflection of deeper changes occurring in the body related to your health or nutritional status (or that physical damage has taken place, such as slamming a nail in a car door, but you'd know about that being the cause!). If your nails aren't what you want them to be or if you've noticed changes in them for reasons you can't explain, consider that they may be a signal from your body that the way you eat, drink, move, think, breathe, believe or perceive needs to change. Nails can, after all, be a reflection of bone health so resolving a nail challenge now may assist bone health in

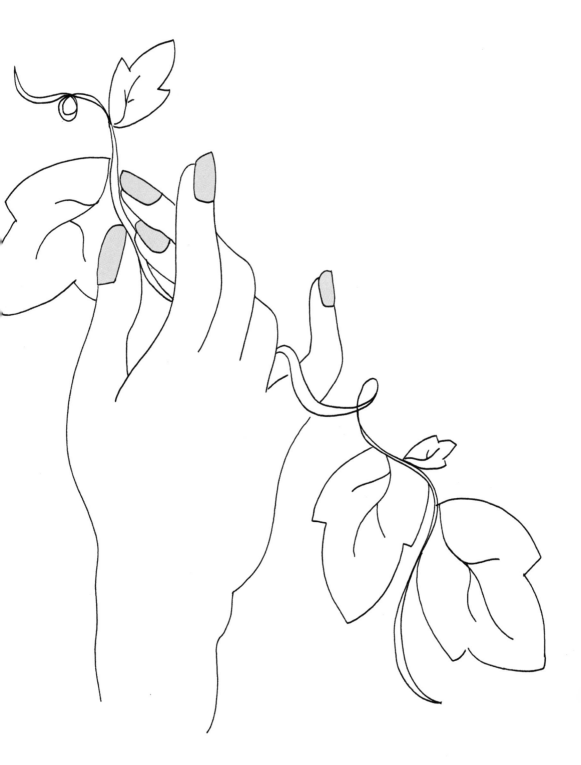

the future. Your nails won't always let you know that your bones are thinning until bone health is significantly compromised (so don't wait for this to happen!), but changes in your nails can mean more bone strengthening nutrients are needed, such as calcium, magnesium, boron and vitamin D.

Nourishment is the key to creating strong, healthy nails. Remember that just because you eat a specific food or nutrient doesn't mean you get it. Much of sparkling health comes down to the way you absorb and utilise nutrients. That being the case, the first step in great quality nails is excellent digestion.

Also, as you will understand in more depth in the upcoming 'Stress' section, nail growth is considered to be a 'non-vital' process, i.e. nails are not necessary to save your life if it was being threatened. So, stress not only takes away from key digestive processes that can impact on nail health, but also the nutrients the nails need are more likely to be used in the creation of stress hormones and other aspects of the get-out-of-danger response than they are to be sent to nourish the nails. Therefore, restorative practices such as tai chi, Stillness Through Movement and restorative yoga—anything that promotes diaphragmatic breathing—fosters the mechanisms that allows your beauty bits, including your nails, to be supported ▣

Tips for Improving Nail Health

Increase your consumption of zinc-rich foods, as white spots on your nails can be a sign you may be zinc deficient. Sources include oysters, red meat, eggs and seeds. You might also like to check out my Bio Blends Zinc, a food-based zinc nutritional supplement.

Peeling cuticles may be an indication of an essential fatty acid (EFA) deficiency. Address this orally while also rubbing a little coconut oil or face oil around your nail beds each evening.

Love your liver! Who would have thought your liver function can be reflected in your nail health? Pale, brittle or weak nails can be an indication that your liver needs some love. Incorporate more of the brassica group of vegetables, such as broccoli, kale and cauliflower.

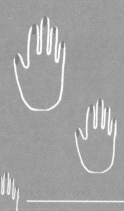

Give your body and nervous system a chance to repair. If your body perceives that it is constantly in danger, the last thing on its list of priorities is maintaining healthy nails.

Do at least one thing every day that is restorative for you, such as yoga, diaphragmatic breathing or simply lying on your back with your legs up the wall for five minutes.

Explore your biochemistry and get some blood tests done, as nail health can be affected by iron deficiency, B12 deficiency or EFA deficiency. EFA tests are only done by specialised labs, while your GP can order iron studies and vitamin B12 blood tests. Refer to page 228 for more details about how these nutrient deficiencies can show up in your nails.

READ MORE

Nail solutions are specifically addressed in the Beauty Solutions section on page 228.

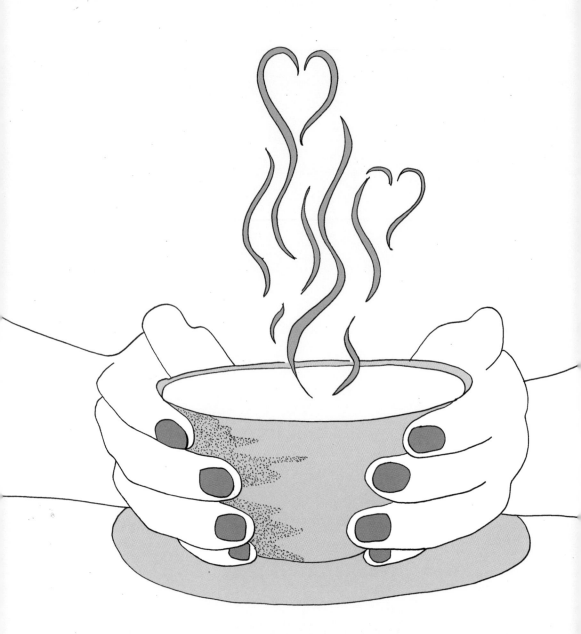

Dr Libby Weaver

Beauty wisdom

Guidance from traditional medicine

In Traditional Chinese Medicine (TCM), luscious locks are attributed to strong kidney energy and what we might think of as robust adrenal function. So, when hair loss is apparent, for example, a TCM practitioner will look to support the vital essence of the kidneys and also treat what they refer to as a blood deficiency. This is not a concept in conventional Western medicine and it doesn't mean you are short on blood—you'd be dead if that was the case!

However, blood does more than just deliver oxygen and nutrients throughout your body. According to TCM principles, blood ensures many tissues are nourished and kept moist and lubricated—think joints, tendons, silky hair and a radiant, even complexion. In TCM, blood deficiency also affects the mind and can lead us to feel scattered, ungrounded, easily stressed out and with poor sleep that can't be explained by other reasons. Think of it that 'strong blood' feels like you are robust, that you can handle challenges—both physical such as a change in the climate or season (you aren't throwing on a jumper at the slightest breeze) as well as mental (in that you feel together and that you can cope when challenges arise). You have a strength and vitality about you and that shows in how you carry yourself, how you communicate as well as via your physical and emotional resilience.

A TCM practitioner will look and listen for the following symptoms of a TCM blood deficiency (1). You don't need to have all of them for there to be a degree of blood deficiency and they will tend to vary in intensity.

THEY INCLUDE*:

- hair that is falling out
- pale-coloured nails, lips and face
- dry skin
- floaters in the visual field (this can be a sign of iron deficiency)
- heavy periods
- tendons that are easily injured
- poor memory and focus
- dizziness
- difficulty falling asleep or staying asleep
- headaches
- migraines
- lack of body strength (you feel 'weak')

So, for not just lustrous hair and skin, and strong nails, but for great health and energy in general, you want to foster great-quality, highly nourishing blood, blood flow and delivery to the tissues.

Please note, these symptoms can be a sign of more serious health conditions so, if you are experiencing any of them, please always consult your GP to rule this out.

Less overthinking: notice when you are worrying about something that may not even happen. Don't worry about something until it is actually a problem. Most things that you worry about don't come to pass.

Do not drink alcohol excessively—only you know if you are doing this. If you feel you can't drink less (in volume or frequency), determine what it is you are seeking for the alcohol to give you (usually a feeling) and work out other ways to obtain this.

HOW CAN YOU BEST SUPPORT A BLOOD-BUILDING LIFESTYLE, ACCORDING TO TCM PRINCIPLES?

Resolve problems with excessive blood loss: if you have heavy menstrual blood loss each month, set out to get answers about why this is occurring. It will almost always involve an excessive amount of estrogen too late in the cycle, something which responds well to dietary changes and liver support. You can read more about this in some of my other books.

If you noticed your health and energy deteriorate after childbirth and you feel like you haven't really ever fully recovered, explore the concept of Postnatal Depletion, coined by Dr Oscar Serrallach (2), who has written a wonderful book called *The Postnatal Depletion Cure.*

Eat regular meals.

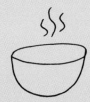

Eat predominantly warm, cooked foods.

Avoid or certainly minimise raw and cold foods including salads, iced drinks, ice-cream and other dairy foods.

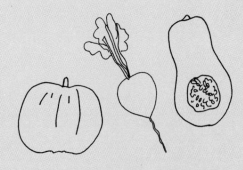

Starchy vegetables, such as pumpkin, sweet potato and beetroot, are highly nourishing for blood deficiency states, as is brown rice.

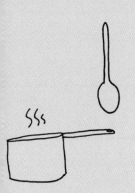

FOOD CONCEPTS TO RECOVER FROM, OR TO HELP PREVENT, TCM BLOOD DEFICIENCY INCLUDE:

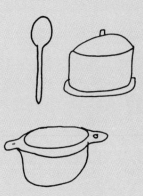

The power of whole, real and, in this case, warm foods is immeasurable.

Nourishing fats such as those found in organic, grass-fed meats, wild-caught fish, organic grass-fed butter, avocado, olives, coconut, nuts and seeds.

Avoid/minimise refined sugars and flours and soy milk in excess.

Bone broth.

Eat plenty of vegetables in the form of soups, stews and casseroles, steamed or stir-fried with some high-quality protein—organic, grass-fed meats or offal (meat cooked on the bone is even better), eggs or lentils.

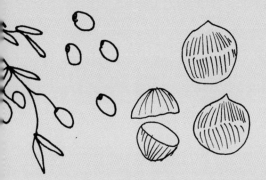

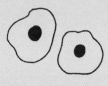

ELIMINAT

&

ON
detoxification

Do you need a detox?

Understanding detoxification and beauty

———

You read everywhere these days that for beautiful skin you need to do a 'detox'. Well, your body is always detoxifying; you wouldn't be here if it wasn't! However, the lifestyle choices you make impact how efficiently the liver and other organs involved in daily detoxification are able to do their critical work.

There is so much misinformation out there about detoxification so let's clear that up.

WHAT IS DETOXIFICATION?

Essentially, it is a change process. Virtually all cells in the body have detoxification actions, but the liver is the main detoxification organ. To keep this simple, I'll focus on the liver.

The liver takes substances that, were they to accumulate, would be harmful to you and converts them into less harmful versions of the original substance in order to be safely eliminated or used for another purpose. For example, alcohol is a poison to the human body. If it were to accumulate in the blood it would be life-threatening, and I don't say that lightly. The liver must change the alcohol into a substance that the body can derive energy (calories) from, to remove it from our circulation. However, in order to do this, it must first convert it into another harmful substance called acetaldehyde. There is only so much the liver is able to convert at once, so if you wake up with a throbbing head after consuming too much alcohol, this is a signal that the liver is struggling to deal with a build-up of acetaldehyde and other problematic substances, such as preservatives in wine.

HOW DOES DETOXIFICATION HAPPEN?

There are two stages to detoxification, known as phase 1 and phase 2. The biochemical reactions of these two phases are driven by specific nutrients. B vitamins and antioxidants, for example, are essential to phase 1, while amino acids and sulphur are critical for phase 2. So, if we are deficient in some (or all) of the nutrients needed as catalysts to these reactions, they won't work as efficiently as they will when we are getting all we need nutritionally. Eat nutrient-dense whole, real foods to give your biochemical pathways what they need to function at their best! Supporting these pathways was a major reason why I formulated Bio Blends Liver Love.

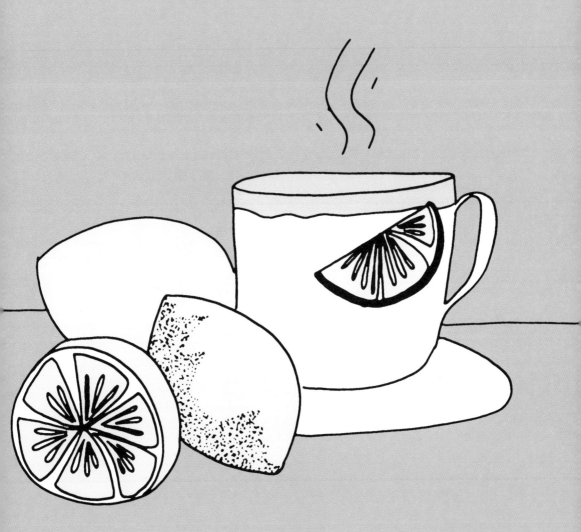

The other important factor to consider in this detox process is: how many 'liver loaders' are going in? For many people today, these need to significantly decrease. Most liver loaders have the potential to slow down the phase 2 reactions—think alcohol, trans fats (found in processed cakes, biscuits and deep-fried foods), certain sugars, synthetic substances (such as pesticides, medications), as well as substances the body makes itself such as cholesterol and estrogen. However, another liver loader, caffeine, speeds up phase 1 and while this might sound exciting (surely something that speeds something up in the body has to be good, right? Not so fast!), it can make things worse for some people.

The best way to picture it is this: if the phase 2 pathways are clear and the traffic on them is flowing, the phase 1 road speeding up will simply result in efficient detoxification. However, for too many people today, traffic on the phase 2 pathways is all banked up like traffic on a motorway, from cumulative poor-quality food and drink choices. If this is the case, when you speed up phase 1, the slightly changed (partially detoxified) substance has no road in phase 2 to transition across to, and it can't stay in the liver as there is always more rubbish coming through the front door.

But your body is incredibly clever, so it has a mechanism through which it can free up space in your liver, while it waits for the traffic jam to clear from the phase 2 pathways. However, this can be cause for concern in the long run, as you'll soon see. Imagine that the liver has a trapdoor and it releases the slightly changed form of the problematic substance back out into the blood supply. This is obviously not ideal since your body sent it to the liver to be detoxified as it wanted it gone from the body, not back in the blood!

The body still has to get this partially detoxified substance—which in some cases is even more reactive or harmful than the original substance—out of the blood, as this is the same blood supply that is going to flow through all of your vital organs. So, the body has another clever alternative solution: the problematic substance is sent to body fat cells to be stored.

This is one of the mechanisms behind cellulite. Not to mention why you might have trouble shifting body fat. Why would the body decide to draw these substances back into the bloodstream if the detoxification pathways are still overwhelmed?

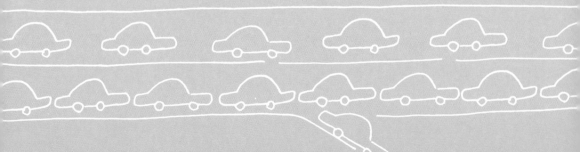

OTHER SIGNS THE LIVER MIGHT BE A LITTLE OVERWHELMED:

- congested skin
- a bloated belly
- a 'liver roll' (a deposit of fat that sits just under the bra-line)
- Premenstrual Syndrome (PMS); heavy, clotty painful periods; mood swings in the lead-up to or during menstruation
- elevated cholesterol

- nausea after eating sometimes
- cellulite
- not hungry for breakfast; you just want coffee
- overheating easily (if this is new for you)
- short temper (if this is new for you).

Eat more brassica vegetables such as broccoli, cauliflower, kale, cabbage and Brussels sprouts.

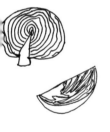

Amp up the whole, real food content of how you eat, particularly plants.

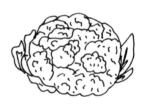

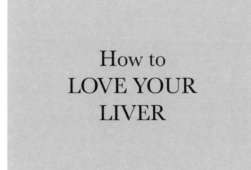

How to LOVE YOUR LIVER

ignificantly reduce
ur intake of refined,
ded sugars (or quit
them entirely).

Minimise liver loaders.

Offer it additional support in the form of medicinal herbs and extracts such as St Mary's thistle, turmeric, globe artichoke, gentian and dandelion root.

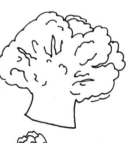

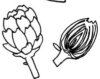

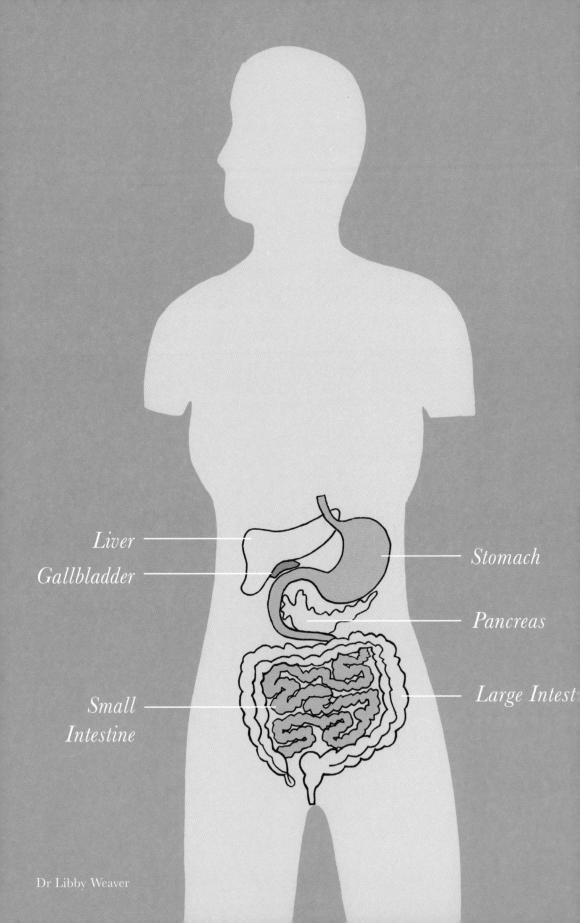

Liver

Gallbladder

Small
Intestine

Stomach

Pancreas

Large Intest

Dr Libby Weaver

The skin-gut connection

Understanding the digestive system

If you want better skin, the place to start is the health and function of your digestive system, as most challenges with the skin originate in the waste-disposal units of the body. If the main routes for waste to leave the body—primarily via the bowels (gut) and the urine (kidneys)—are overloaded or inefficient, the skin will put its hand up and step in to allow the waste to leave that way.

It is important to remember, though, that, like everything, the digestive system doesn't work alone. It requires the optimal function of its ancillary organs as well as its own good function for you to reap the rewards of clear skin. The ancillary organs to the digestive system include the liver, the gallbladder and the pancreas.

All of this means that sometimes skin challenges will be related to something specific about the gut that needs to be addressed, such as stomach acid production, stress reduction to improve the blood flow to the gut as well as decreasing intestinal permeability (aka 'leaky gut'), altering gut pH, or getting rid of unwanted bugs (such as parasites) that have taken up residence somewhere they are not supposed to be. Other times, it is the liver or the production of bile (stored in the gallbladder) that need the attention. Let's explore these in more detail.

THE DIGESTIVE SYSTEM

The best way to picture the digestive tract is as a long tube that begins in your mouth and ends where the waste leaves your body. Food enters your mouth—you are supposed to chew it, not inhale it— and it then continues its journey down your oesophagus into the stomach, where hydrochloric acid is released. The job of this acid is to continue the work of the teeth in breaking the food down. Good stomach acid production also helps to establish what is known as the pH gradient of the gut. This means that the ideal pH for each region of the digestive tract gradually increases from being very acidic in the stomach to almost neutral when the waste leaves you via your faeces. This is critical to the optimal function of the whole digestive system as, if the pH is not ideal in a particular area of the large intestine, for example, nasty bugs can take up residence there. If the pH was ideal, the bad bugs couldn't survive there and build their camps.

HOW DO YOU BEST SUPPORT THE STOMACH ACID TO DO ITS CRITICAL WORK?

1. Eat slowly and chew your food really well as chewing sends a message to the brain to tell the stomach to release its acid.

2. Drink water between meals, not with meals, as the pH of the acid is about 1.9, while the pH of water is 7 or greater. If you drink with meals, you risk diluting the stomach acid, interfering with its ability to do its vital work.

3. Stimulate stomach acid production by drinking apple cider vinegar or lemon juice in warm water before meals: either breakfast or meals rich in protein.

The small intestine is where almost all the vitamins and minerals in your food move from your digestive system across into your blood.

This is how you are nourished, and this process of absorption is essential to your survival. If this didn't work, life would end! This is how all the cells and tissues, including the skin, obtain the nutrients they need to be their best from the blood.

HOW DO YOU BEST SUPPORT NUTRIENT ABSORPTION FROM THE SMALL INTESTINE?

1. Eat nutrient-dense food so you actually have something to absorb! If you eat too many poor-quality, packaged, processed foods and takeaways, the levels of nutrients available for all of these critical processes will be compromised.

2. Good absorption relies on the right pH, so supporting good stomach acid production is vital to the small intestine being able to do its critical absorption work.

3. If you consume coffee or tea, don't drink it for at least 30 minutes either side of eating as they can block the absorption of a range of nutrients due to their caffeine and tannin content.

4. Iron and calcium compete for absorption and iron deficiency is the most common nutritional deficiency in the world, particularly among women of menstruation age. It is therefore best to eat iron-rich foods away from calcium-rich foods, to maximise your absorption of both. In other words, don't drink a glass of milk with or immediately after you eat a steak or you may obtain very little iron from the steak.

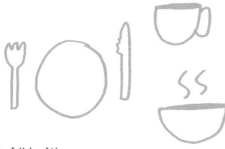

Dr Libby Weaver

THE LARGE INTESTINE

The large intestine plays a host of different roles in your health along with what's happening on the outside. To keep this simple, imagine the bacteria that live in here are programmed to ferment whatever is delivered to them. They can handle receiving food that is pretty well broken down by all of the processes that have gone on before now. But if something has gone awry in an earlier aspect of digestion, the bacteria will receive fragments of food too large for them to handle effectively. They will still try to ferment it, but the by-product of this is often excessive or uncomfortable gas, leading to bloating and/or excessive or odorous flatulence. When people think of bloating they often think there must be something wrong with their large intestine, yet you can see that if what I've just described is occurring, it is due to processes further up the digestive system.

The next thing to consider is that unfavourable bugs can take up residence in the large intestine due to the pH not being hospitable to the beneficial species you want living there. Or you may have travelled and had food poisoning or picked up something from the water supply or via water that is used to wash food, for example. These 'parasites' can set up residence in the large intestine and lead to bloating, irritable bowel-type symptoms and a tummy that sounds very gurgly.

For myriad reasons, people experience constipation or diarrhoea, or intermittent bouts of both. Presenting every last reason for this is beyond the scope of this book, but please consider which of the processes described here may not be working efficiently in you and that might be leading to these symptoms. Apply what you are learning and don't give up until you have great gut function, formed stools and use your bowels every day.

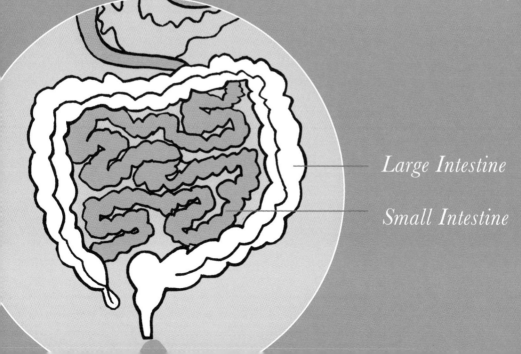

Large Intestine

Small Intestine

HOW DO YOU BEGIN TO ADDRESS THESE CHALLENGES?

1. Apply the stomach acid support strategies from earlier in this piece to help ensure that the fermenting bacteria only receive fragments of food they can handle.

2. If your gut challenges were initiated by a travel experience, you may need to deal with parasites. Herbs that can be useful for this include Chinese wormwood and black walnut, but it's best to consult with a qualified health professional who can guide you with this.

3. Dietary changes are sometimes necessary for gut function to improve. Common dietary trials that may prove beneficial include ones without gluten (found in wheat, rye, barley, oats and triticale), casein (found in all dairy foods and processed foods that have had dairy products added to them), or a low/modified FODMAP way of eating (which decreases the fermentable components of your dietary intake). It goes without saying that you first want to omit all artificial substances from how you eat: sweeteners, flavours, additives and preservatives. Any dietary changes are best guided by an experienced nutrition professional.

THE ROLE STRESS PLAYS

Stress reduction to improve blood flow to the digestive system and decrease intestinal permeability can be a vital step in improving gut function and hence the appearance of the skin. When we have elevated levels of stress hormones, the fight or flight response—driven by the activation of the sympathetic nervous system (SNS)—promotes blood flow away from the digestive system to the periphery (to the arms and the legs) as this is what is going to give you the best chance at escaping from the impending danger your body thinks you are in. In other words, stress can significantly compromise digestion.

Stress hormones also promote increased intestinal permeability—known these days as 'leaky gut'—as they create larger gaps between the cells that line the intestines. This means that food that is not fully broken down can end up in the blood, promoting an immune response as well as inflammation. Only nutrients (not foods) are supposed to end up in the blood.

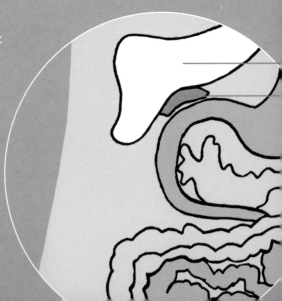

How do you decrease the constant, relentless output of stress hormones that so many people experience these days?

Refer to page 146 for a comprehensive list of suggestions.

LOVE YOUR LIVER

Showing your liver some more love can be an essential step in improving skin clarity, particularly if you have constant or recurring pimples or acne. Why this important is explained in the article on page 59. For many people, including those with skin problems that began at puberty, or are sex hormone-related, liver support can be the game changer.

How do you better support your liver?

Embrace the strategies outlined on page 91.

THE GALLBLADDER AND BILE

The gallbladder stores the bile that the liver makes. If you have had yours surgically removed, the liver has to make bile on demand. Bile is needed to prepare fatty substances for detoxification by the liver. Your own sex hormones, as well as pesticides, are all fat-soluble substances that require

altering before they can be excreted. If bile production is inefficient, this can lead these problematic substances to remain too long in the body. The best way to think about this is that these hovering substances cause congestion—congestion on the roads leading into the liver, as well as congestion in your skin (refer to page 90 for more on this).

How do you promote good bile production?

1. Bitter foods which include green leafy vegetables and some herbs such as dandelion root (think dandelion tea).

2. Ensure good stomach acid production using the aforementioned tips, including chewing your food well.

3. Medicinal herbs such as globe artichoke, St Mary's thistle and gentian, which is one of the many reasons I included them in Bio Blends Liver Love.

This is a snapshot of these miraculous processes that work so hard to keep you looking and feeling your best. Do all you can to help them do what they were born to do, which is to help keep you nourished and the waste efficiently transformed and released ■

—— Liver

—— Gallbladder

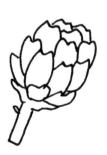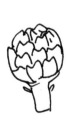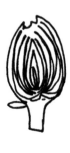

When your skin becomes an exit ramp

The skin's role in eliminating toxins

———

When the skin is asking for your attention—which it does via signs and symptoms that you find challenging—the first port of call must be to examine the efficiency of the elimination and detoxification processes as, along with its many other roles, the skin is part of that system.

The main roads of elimination of waste out of the body are via the bowels and urine. For the gut to do its job properly, the detoxification pathways of the liver must do their critical work preparing some substances for elimination in the stools. And the kidneys must filter the blood to create urine so waste can also exit the body this way.

The skin offers another road out of the body for waste, but you don't want to have to ask it to step in to do this, other than through sweating. You don't want it to become congested or inflamed due to other waste products not finding their way out via the bowels and the urine. You want your skin to be the radiant protective organ it is supposed to be.

WHEN MIGHT THE SKIN STEP IN?

Put simply, if too many problematic substances enter your body via what you eat, drink, breathe or put on your skin, or if your body is getting the message to (internally) produce excessive amounts of substances that the liver will have to change before you can excrete them (think cholesterol and estrogen) then the preferred exits from the body may not be able to keep up with their loads. Yet, the waste has to leave somehow, so the skin steps in to help out.

Another reason why the skin may need to assist in the removal of waste from the body is if the nutrients needed to make the detoxification and elimination pathways run efficiently are not available because you haven't eaten enough of them. Think too many processed foods devoid of nutrients, not enough vegetables, or simply not eating enough full stop. Or it may be because the body is busy sending nutrients off to be used in the 'saving your life' processes that stress hormones communicate are a priority, and there aren't enough left over for the biochemical pathways linked to detoxification.

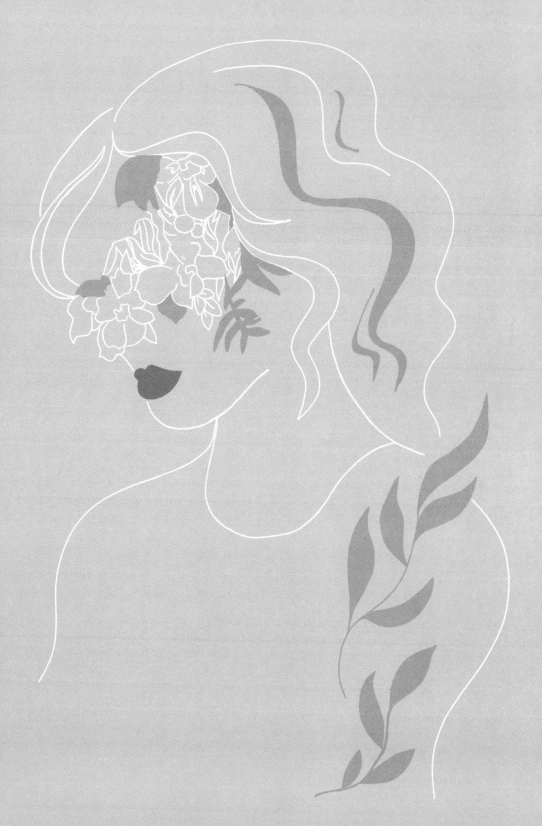

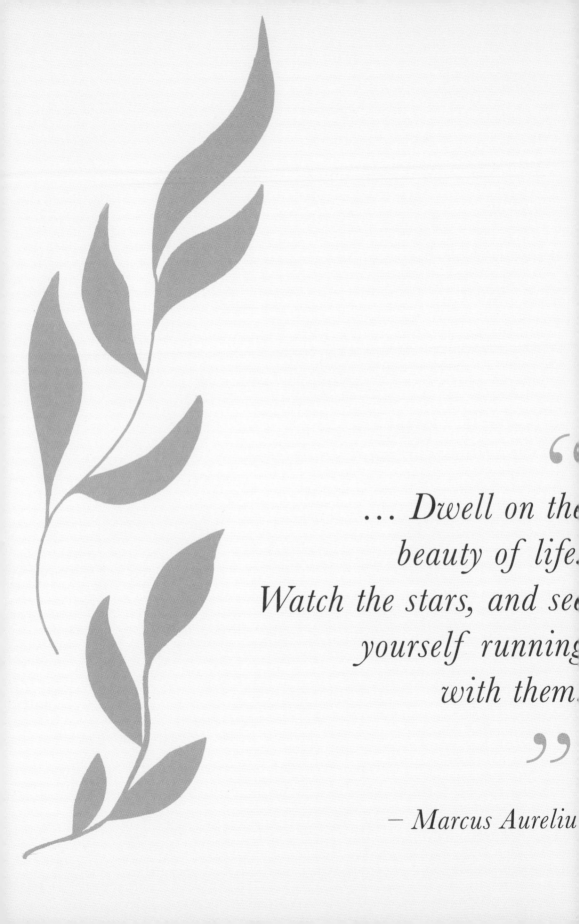

"... Dwell on the beauty of life. Watch the stars, and see yourself running with them."

— Marcus Aureliu

REDNESS

CYSTS UNDER
THE SKIN OR
BREAKING
THROUGH
THE SKIN

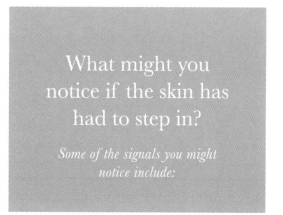
What might you notice if the skin has had to step in?

Some of the signals you might notice include:

CONGESTION
UMPS UNDER
E SKIN; SKIN IS
OT SMOOTH)

ACNE

PIMPLES

BREAKOUTS RELATED TO
YOUR MENSTRUAL CYCLE

o prevent the skin having to step in as a pathway of elimination from the body n a way that could feel challenging for ou, consider how you can best support ll of these elimination, detoxification nd filtration systems to work at their est. Instead of being frustrated with our skin, think of it as a mechanism of ommunication for you to take even etter care of your digestive system, liver nd kidneys. Think of any problems you otice on your skin as a reminder to you o eat more whole, real foods and fewer or no) processed foods. Also, make water our main drink. See it as an opportunity o learn about a way of life that better upports your own great health and nergy, as well as that of the planet.

t is wonderful to do what we can to ninimise the problematic substances that nter our body. Some of these we can't

control, like the exhaust from the number of cars on the road, while others we can influence, such as pesticide consumption or exposure to the synthetic chemicals used in conventional household cleaning products and skincare. In my experience, there are two camps when it comes to this situation: there are those people who stress about every last thing they might have been exposed to and see 'toxins' in everything. And the opposite end of that spectrum falls to those who have little or no awareness of their exposures. Or if they do, they don't act to minimise them. So, a good thing to focus on for both groups is how we best support our body to efficiently eliminate what we are exposed to. For health might only be compromised if the problematic substances accumulate, rather than get eliminated ■

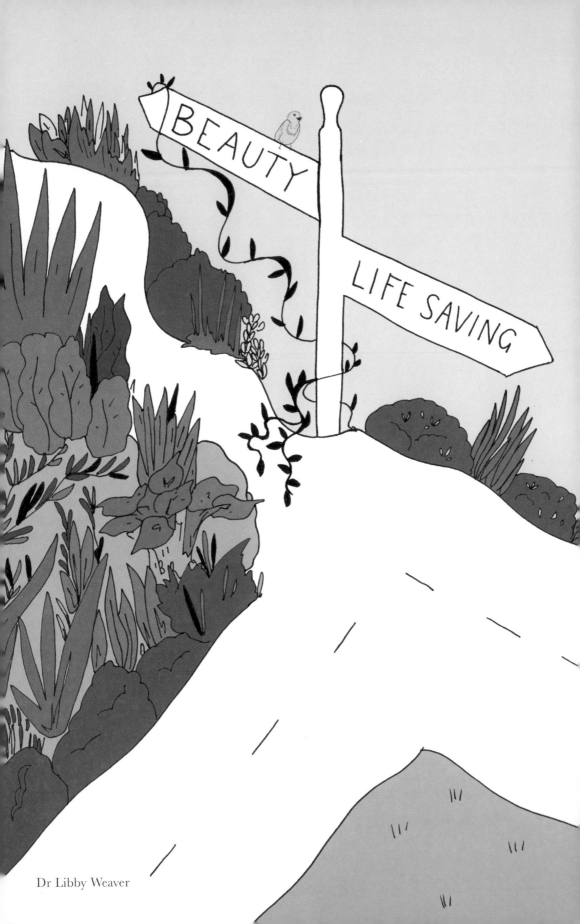

Dr Libby Weaver

Why beauty ranks last

How your body prioritises

Your liver doesn't just do miraculous detoxification work. It also helps to distribute nutrients throughout your body to where they are most needed. These processes have a ranking system—and your survival is highest on the list. This is why beauty bits can miss out when you are living on stress hormones, for example, as your survival always has to come first.

THE BEST WAY TO PICTURE IT IS THIS...

You eat a meal that is rich in calcium. You (hopefully) chew it well and your digestive system extracts the calcium from the food as part of the breakdown process. This calcium is absorbed across the intestinal wall into the blood. This nutrient-rich blood then travels to the liver. The liver scans your body for where this calcium is most needed.

When you think of where calcium is best utilised in your body, what do you think of? Bones usually? Or teeth. Yet you could survive if both of these structures were in lousy shape. You could break multiple bones and still be alive.

The first place the calcium must be maintained for you to stay alive is in your blood. Your blood level of calcium is essential to life, while the strength of your bones or teeth isn't.

After the blood and countless other biochemical processes and cellular needs have been met, there is (hopefully) some calcium left over for your bones. And your teeth. Your nails need calcium for their strength too. Yet let's say, when the liver receives this influx of calcium, it scans your body and can see that the little fingernail on your right hand is wearing a bit thin and is in need of some calcium. If there is actually any calcium left over after meeting the needs of all of these other processes, the liver will program some units of calcium and send them to your nails. Doesn't that blow your mind?

YOUR BODY WILL ALWAYS FOCUS ON SAVING YOUR LIFE OVER HOW YOU LOOK.

However, I want you to appreciate that for there to be any nutrients left over for your beauty bits, you have to consume enough of them in the first place. This is what I mean by beauty ranks last ∎

The fear of holding on

A case study

———

Note, the following pages contain information about purging behaviours. If this may be triggering for you, please feel free to skip to the next section.

She was 16 years old when they said it: 'There goes a big girl'. When little boys point to a teenager and make that comment, what do you think they mean by 'big'? Taller? Older? Of course. The meaning she created was that 'even the little kids think I'm fat'. And so began the story of one of the most challenging patients I ever worked with.

From that point forward she started restricting her food intake. 'I'll only eat brown rice and broccoli for dinner', and she'd only allow herself the rice if she'd run the 10km track she'd mapped out after school. Every last morsel that passed her lips was calculated.

Her health began to suffer, she lost her energy and her glow, and her hair started falling out.

The next year, she was sent away to boarding school and was confronted with the food on offer. She'd always lived at home until now. At first she avoided as much of it as she could, and this is when her bowels stopped working efficiently for the first time. Her diary shows that she'd go eight days sometimes without using them. But this was the first time she recounts that the concept of 'toxins'

accumulating occurred to her and she grew worried that not pooing would make her gain weight. She started to eat a little more and this helped her bowels a little, but she was still only going about twice a week on average.

———

EVERY LAST MORSEL THAT PASSED HER LIPS WAS CALCULATED.

———

So she started eating more, but her bowels still wouldn't move daily the way they once had. She'd heard about laxatives and thought she might need them. At first they didn't do much, so she took more and more, until finally her bowels really let go.

Over the coming weeks she shared that she 'fell in love with the feeling of having diarrhoea each day'. This is because she thought it would lead to weight loss to compensate for how much more she was eating these days (most of which was very poor-quality food).

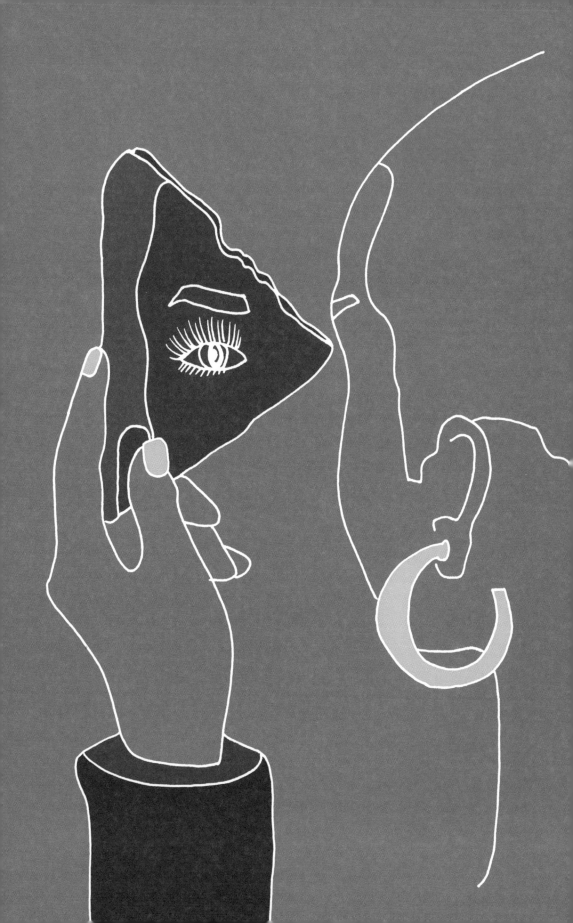

Once she returned home and back to her old school, she told me how she would start eating and feel like she couldn't stop. Her answer to this was to use laxatives to not freak out that she'd gain weight. Her vicious cycle was continuing.

Then one night at a party, her boyfriend reached out to her to put his hands on her waist and she wriggled away, which led him to say, 'I used to love to touch you there.' She interpreted this as 'even he thinks I'm fat now', and it sent her into an even deeper cycle of eating and trying to get rid of the waste. Getting rid of the waste became her attempted weight loss strategy now that she felt she couldn't control her appetite or restrict her food intake enough to be as slim as she wanted to be.

What she didn't realise was the laxatives were contributing to the confused messages her body was getting about whether to burn body fat as a fuel. This meant her body fat did the opposite of what she thought the laxatives would do and she stored more fat instead.

This dear girl got well over time—healed her bowel and her relationship with food, but I share this part of her story with you as it was the first time I really witnessed the bowels being used in an attempt to control weight.

Of course, I've seen this plenty of times since—women use all sorts of things to make their bowels move so that they feel thinner, which is a short-term feeling that can lead to longer term damage. I hear many younger women talking about how they need to do yet another 'cleanse' to get rid of the 'toxins' that have built up.

> *I HEAR MANY YOUNGER WOMEN TALKING ABOUT HOW THEY NEED TO DO YET ANOTHER 'CLEANSE' TO GET RID OF THE 'TOXINS' THAT HAVE BUILT UP.*

Now don't get me wrong, there are times when this approach might be warranted. With a fatty liver, for example, incorporating more vegetables and vegie juices into the diet can be a marvellous stepping stone to instigate change and improvements. But in this case, the young women I'm referring to aren't being medically guided to do their fifth cleanse for the year and it usually doesn't suit their body composition as they are often already blood deficient (to use the TCM description) and have poor muscle mass.

They are cold and don't have robust health. They use less food or only juices and extra bowel motions as a body-control mechanism, sadly motivated by fear, not health. Fear of weight gain, fear of toxins, fear of... themselves and their

wn appetites… of everything. They are
sually fearful of change, yet experience
he irony of wanting it all to speed
p—their bowels, their body tone, their
uccess in life.

lease know that focusing on supporting
our body to detoxify and eliminate
roblematic substances as efficiently as
ossible isn't the issue here—I'm not
enying our world isn't polluted and that
he body needs additional support these
ays. But you can do this with a genuine
ocus and motivation that stems from
ealth rather than from fear. And only you
now which one it truly is for you.

So live a lifestyle that allows you to use
your bowels each day, with a focus on
health. If you can recognise that you've
been making choices from fear, not love
(of your dear self or your health), do
what you can or seek help to assist you
to change this. It is possible to have a
deeply appreciative relationship with your
Earth Suit, nourishing it and allowing it to
get rid of waste, without you having to
stress about it. And the first step on that
road is to truly feel the beauty of your
own soul ■

*For additional support, please refer to the
Resources on page 263.*

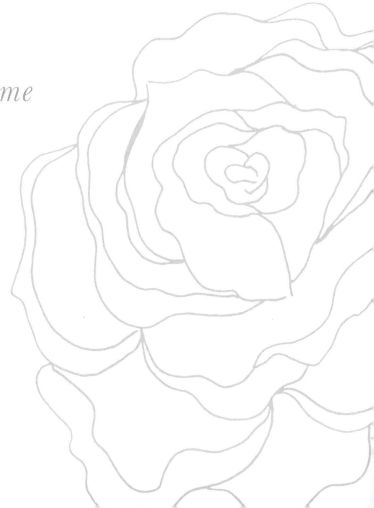

*'And the day came
when the risk to
remain tight in
a bud was more
painful than
the risk it took
to blossom.'*

- Anais Nin

STR

ESS

What do you hide

UNDER THE COVER OF STRESS?

What most people worry about is what other people think of them.

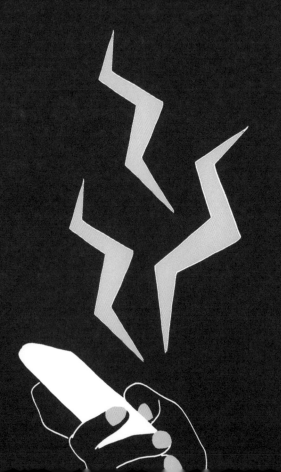
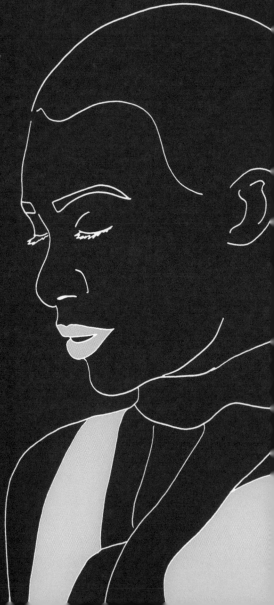

What are you really stressed about?

Pulling back the covers

The mechanisms behind the stress response drive degeneration—what we refer to as ageing. So rather than simply wishing that life was less stressful—which feels like a pipe dream for many—let's explore what gets us into this state. Now that you have an understanding of the way that stress hormones compromise the non-essential beauty processes (refer to page 103), consider your own stresses and what you feel pressure and urgency about in your own life.

WHAT IS STRESS?

What is stress, really? It is a word we use so easily and often without much thought these days. Not that long ago in human evolution it would have meant that our life was threatened. Now we report feeling stressed about our to-do lists, email inboxes and running late. Stress can also refer to trauma and the after-effects of this can lead to a continued stress response for some people. Please note that, in this piece, I am not referring to trauma but rather the everyday stresses that people describe.

In my opinion, stress is the achiever's word for fear. It's just that it would sound quite odd to tell people that you are scared of your emails (although you may have joked about this at times!). Think about the last time you felt really worked up on the inside. You may not have shown this outwardly to anyone, but you were stressed. Let's say it was because you were running late for a meeting. Pause to consider what the stress might really have been about. Consider it this way: 'If stress is actually showing me something that I'm frightened of, what might that be?' And what you'll see when you pull the veil back on what stresses you out—in this case the 'running late'—what most people are scared of is what other people think of them.

Once you see the stress for what it really is, you can decide if you stay in that worked-up state or not, as now you can see the truth: you aren't stressed, you are worried about what someone (or a group of people) thinks of you. With this insight, you can pause and think through what's really bothering you about this scenario instead of futilely repeating over and over again in your mind 'I'm so stressed, I'm so stressed'. What are you worried that they'll think of you? How are you concerned that they will perceive you? Name the traits.

Each individual has constructed an identity. And we will do anything to stay true to that identity. I describe it this way at my women's weekend events:

You have a word written across your forehead and it is so important to you that people view you in this way. You will do anything to remain congruent with that word, including sacrificing your own health (a concept I discuss in my book *Rushing Woman's Syndrome*).

So, when you run late and that stresses you out (remember it doesn't stress everyone out), what character traits are you worried will be applied to you?

And are they the opposite of how you want to be seen?

What word is drawn across your forehead? What traits are important to you and how do you prefer to be seen? Name them. Here are some common examples that people have shared with me over the years…

STRONG

RESPECTFUL

PERFECT

SELFLESS

THOUGHTFUL

KIND

CONSIDERATE

LOVELY

HELPFUL

HONEST

INDEPENDENT

Dr Libby Weaver

ou might like to take this a step further. When did this trait (or these traits) in you rst begin? Do you recall? They usually evelop in response to you trying to lease a parent. We develop these parts f our personality when we are very oung, unconsciously in the pursuit of anting to remain safe. And safety when ou are six years old means being loved y your parent/s, because you would find impossible to independently take care f yourself at that age.

Vhat arises when you ponder this? For nany, they start to see how parts of their ersonality have been constructed in esponse to the fear that they are not nough unless they behave in a certain ay. As opposed to just being who they re (as I outlined in the Introduction). So e develop these masks that we wear. nd we feel like we need to keep it lastered in place so that people (now hat you are older, it's often all people, r certainly a wider circle of people, not ust your parents) see you in this way. Our rive to remain congruent to our identity very, very powerful.

his part of the puzzle became apparent o me when I started to work with more omen in a younger age bracket. I'd sk them what stresses them out and ney'd say 'my Instagram posts'. They'd ell me sometimes they are in tears after osting something, worrying that they'll e judged or that people will notice their laws'. Others feel the 'pressure' to post nany times a day and not having the ontent' stresses them out enormously.

In all honesty, I couldn't understand this at first, yet the young women in front of me were clearly stressed out about it. Whereas women of my generation and older tend to rush, worried that they'll let someone down or not be able to do the juggling act of work and family as well as they'd like to, ensuring everyone feels valued and loved. It's just two different ways this same pattern plays out and at different life stages.

So next time you find yourself stressing out on the inside, pause and ask yourself with the gentle tenderness you would approach a child with: 'If this is truly something I'm frightened of, what might it be?' And you'll see who you are trying to please and who you worry about when it comes to how they see you. And I hope in that moment you see how futile and unnecessary and, at times, damaging this is.

YOU DON'T HAVE TO ACT A CERTAIN WAY FOR PEOPLE TO LOVE AND APPRECIATE YOU.

You just need to be you—your authentic self. And with the truth of all this, you'll find a new way to live. With far less 'stress' and all of the benefits inside and out that that brings ∎

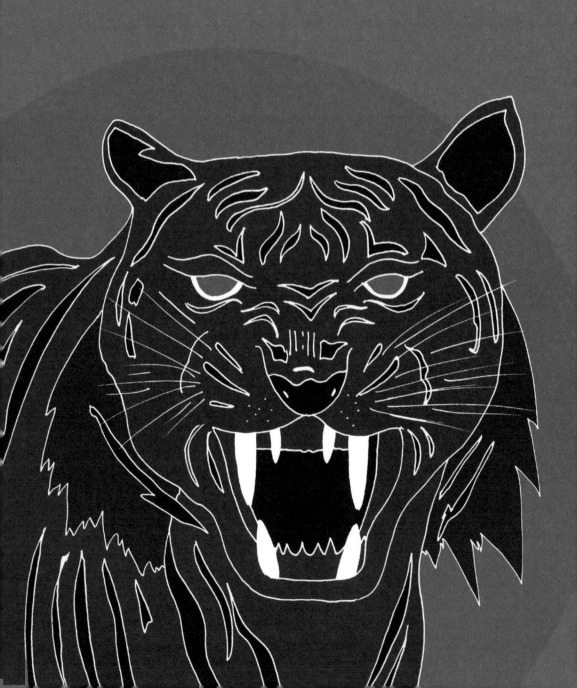

Beauty and your survival

Why the outside may suffer

Your body will do anything to keep you alive. It has your survival at its heart. This means, however, that the production of stress hormones and other vital processes are considered to be far more essential than how strong your nails are. Here's how it works.

The adrenal glands (which sit just on top of each of your kidneys) make a wide variety of substances, including your stress hormones—adrenaline and cortisol. For the very long time that humans have been on the planet (think 150,000 to 200,000 years), adrenaline, what you may know as the 'fight or flight' hormone, has communicated to every cell in our body that our life is literally in danger. Because, historically, the only time we made it was when this was the case. However, in modern times, disregarding any situation where our life might actually be in danger, there are new and different things that lead the body to get the message that it needs to produce adrenaline—many of which occur on a daily basis.

For example, we produce adrenaline when we consume anything that contains caffeine (sorry, but it's true!), and our coffee culture means that, for the vast majority of people, coffee has become a daily habit. But the real change has taken place in the increase of psychological stress. What I mean by this is that our body can get the message to produce adrenaline based on something as simple as our perception of pressure and urgency.

So many people have forgotten that they get to choose how they see their day!

NEVER LOSE SIGHT OF HOW PRIVILEGED WE ARE BECAUSE ALL OF OUR BASIC NEEDS ARE MET, WHEN FOR SO MANY PEOPLE IN THE WORLD THEY AREN'T.

This isn't to say there aren't stressful things in your world, it's only to serve as a reminder that our perception can make a huge difference to how we feel about our lives.

The body has not yet evolved to be able to discern between the adrenaline you make when your life is in danger, such as when a car drives out in front of you unexpectedly and you have to slam on your brakes, and the adrenaline you make because you've had a few coffees and have 200 unopened emails that you have no idea where you're going to find the time to respond to. To the body it is all the same: danger. And to help you escape from danger, adrenaline drives a host of biochemical changes inside you.

Your blood pressure increases, blood is diverted away from supporting great digestion to the periphery (think your arms and legs) to help you fight or flee. Plus, this elevation in your adrenaline levels tells your body that you need a fast-burning fuel to help you escape from the danger you are supposedly in.

THERE ARE ONLY TWO FUELS FOR THE HUMAN BODY—GLUCOSE AND FAT. IN ANY GIVEN MOMENT WE ARE TYPICALLY USING A COMBINATION OF BOTH.

When your body is getting the message that your life is in danger, it needs a fast-burning fuel to get you out of that danger. So take a wild guess which is your fast-burning fuel? Glucose. Your body believes it has more chance of survival if it supplies you with predominantly glucose

and, as a result, your ability to use body fat as a fuel can become compromised. Plus, you will likely crave sweet food to top up your diminishing stores.

Cortisol is our chronic stress hormone. Historically, chronic stress was typically due to floods, famines and/or wars. If you think about each of these scenarios, food was scarce. So when we produce it today due to modern-day chronic stressors such as relationship concerns, financial concerns, worries about school/university grades or friends, what we look like, what other people think of us, health concerns, the health concerns of a loved one, or weight—whatever is always on your mind—the body still thinks that food is scarce.

In order to save your life in these situations, one of cortisol's jobs is to slow your metabolic rate down and it does this by breaking down your muscles. Not just the muscles that are visible on the outside such as your biceps, but also structural muscles that hold your organs in place and those needed to keep skin taut. More on the skin-related consequences of this shortly. For now, simply consider that when you have less muscle mass, your metabolic rate slows down. Historically, it made sense for your body to do this as the more body fat you could hang on to, the more likely you were to survive the famine that you were supposedly part of

Always remember
THAT YOU GET TO *CHOOSE* HOW YOU SEE YOUR DAY.

In modern times, this mechanism typically leads to much frustration as clothes become tight for no 'obvious' reasons related to food intake and movement patterns.

You may be wondering why your body can't just get with the program and learn to distinguish the difference between real danger and your troubled thoughts about your to-do list, bills and deadlines. Well, unfortunately, evolution just doesn't work that way. We're not computers and we can't just insert new software that brings us up to speed! Evolutionary changes take place gradually from generation to generation; much slower than the pace of change we've seen over the last 100–200 years—not to mention the last 20 years. So until our biochemistry catches up (which is not going to happen within our lifetime!), we need to take into consideration the way we are built and do what we can to support our biochemistry to not interpret danger every single day.

For every unit of adrenaline and cortisol you make you need a range of nutrients, including B vitamins, vitamin C and magnesium. But here's the catch. You also need vitamin C to prevent the breakdown of collagen and to produce new collagen for your skin. And you need magnesium for strong bones and nails. So if these nutrients are in limited supply because you don't consume enough of them to meet all of your needs through eating too much processed food, or if you are going through a particularly stressful time and making more adrenaline than you usually would, your skin and nail health and overall appearance will be compromised. Because your body has to save your life first.

Furthermore, the stress response is one reason why cellulite creeps in. The liver is involved in this too. So how does it happen?

As you learnt on page 52, the skin is made up of three layers and at the bottom of the third layer—the subcutaneous layer—muscle supports the structure and appearance of the top layer of skin. Remember that from the age of 30 onwards, we gradually lose muscle mass from throughout our whole body, unless we actively do something to combat this.

Add to this natural decline in muscle mass the loss that occurs when excessive amounts of cortisol are made (for whom is it not made these days?), and you create space for fat to infiltrate this third layer of skin. The best way to picture it is this: when a muscle shrinks in size, a space is formed where once the muscle filled. Such gaps invite the liver loaders that couldn't be fully transformed (detoxified—refer to page 88 to recap on this) to be wrapped up in fat and deposited here as it is considered a safe space—safe because the problematic substances are being housed away from the vital organs that keep you alive. So you can see that a common pathway to cellulite is due to muscle loss, stress and liver congestion ∎

> Here's a common scenario I've seen hundreds, if not thousands of times in both adult women and teenagers...

1 A diet that is based mostly on processed, packaged foods or takeaways

2 Main drink is not water

3 Stress creeps in over time and nutrient deficiencies such as iron and zinc become more pronounced, hair starts falling out so hair extensions are added to thicken it up

4 Congested skin (face and/or chest and back) or acne with a belief that a different skincare routine is the answer

5 Cellulite appears and gets worse over time, whether there is evidence of high levels of body fat or not

6 Nails hardly grow and if they do, they are weak, soft or ridged and break easily so false nails are applied to cover them up

These scenarios are predominantly due to poor nutrition, stress and a liver that has a lot of work to do. All three of these factors mess with sex hormones as well, which then have their own impact on the beauty bits. Not to mention that the body's ability to repair and protect itself is also compromised.

> So how do we begin
> to unravel this?

1

Build muscle:

- Resistance training, yoga and Pilates all help you to build muscle.

- Don't avoid movement, particularly weight-bearing movement: carry your luggage, your groceries and your children.

- Do gardening or farm work.

- Use your body; don't shy away from movement.

- Stand rather than sit for your work day.

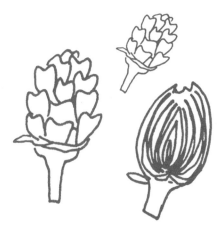

2

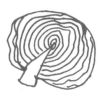

Nutrients:

- Maximise nutrient intake and minimise the intake of artificial substances.

- Eat in a way that is based on whole, real food, minimal processed food and make water your main drink.

3

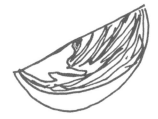

Support the liver:

- Strategies for this are offered on page 91.

4 Lower stress hormones:

- Decrease caffeine so you make less adrenaline.
- Explore your perceptions of what is urgent and full of pressure in your life.

Swap 'I have to' for 'I get to' when you look at your to-do list.

Consider if your stress is really related to you worrying about what other people think of you, explored more on page 111 and see if you can therefore see this situation with new eyes.

- Become breath aware and embrace a breath-focused practice such as tai chi, Stillness Through Movement, meditation, restorative yoga or simply commit to doing 20 long, slow breaths at predetermined intervals across the day such as when you are at red traffic lights, every hour on the hour if you have a desk job, on waking or on going to bed.

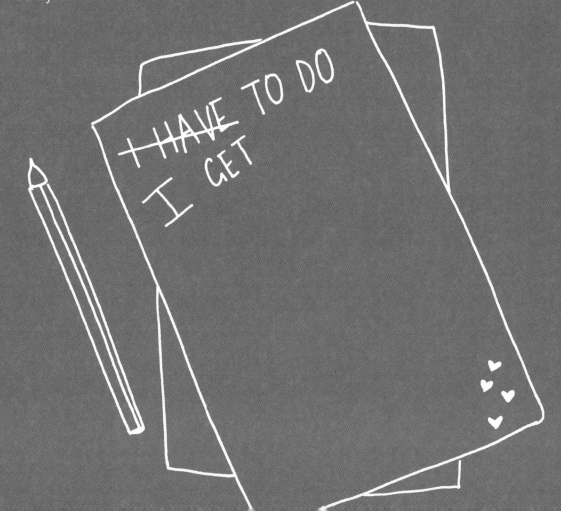

I HAVE TO DO
I GET

The mother gland

How your body is wired for safety

———

Feeling safe—physically and emotionally—is vital to our health. If we don't feel safe, knowingly or unknowingly, it can result in the stress response being switched on more often than it is off. And this can take an immense toll on our inner health, our sleep, as well as what reflects on the outside.

HERE'S HOW THE CONCEPT OF SAFETY WORKS INSIDE YOUR BODY:

In the middle of your brain sits the hypothalamus, the master control switch for your whole endocrine system (the assortment of glands that make hormones throughout your body). Among other important tasks, it asks 24/7: 'Am I safe?'

It makes that assessment via two predominant fields: the physical and the emotional. Based on the response it receives (a distinct 'yes' or 'no'; there is no grey area with 'safety' in the body), the hypothalamus then communicates to the pituitary gland—I call her the 'mother gland'—whether you are indeed safe or not. She then sends out her signals based on whether she received information about your safety or a lack thereof.

That means that your adrenal glands (where you make stress hormones, some sex hormones, as well as blood pressure-regulating hormones, just to name a few), thyroid, ovaries, parts of your digestive system and even your body fat, then make their hormones to suit your 'conditions', i.e. whether you are safe or not.

So let's back up the bus and work out how your body gets the message that you are safe or not.

ON A PHYSICAL LEVEL

When the hypothalamus asks, 'Am I safe?', it looks to the rest of your nervous system for input, including the parts involved in fear and emotions. All day, every day, your nervous system is monitoring and relaying to the hypothalamus information about your internal organs, what you can see and smell, the nutrient and energy stores in your body, and the amount of stress hormones that are circulating in your blood. As you already understand, adrenaline communicates to every cell in your body that your life is in danger so when it is present, the feedback to the hypothalamus is immediately

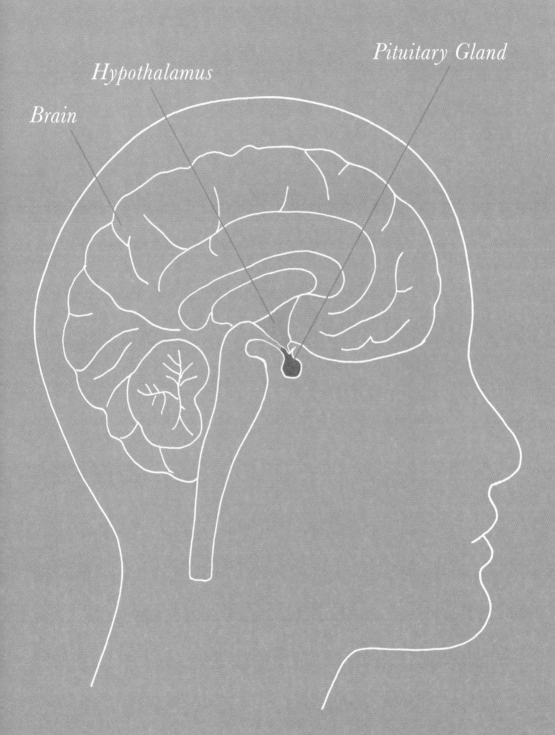

Brain

Hypothalamus

Pituitary Gland

HOW MANY DAYS
DO YOU SPEND
WITH ELEVATED
ADRENALINE DUE
TO YOUR CAFFEINE
CONSUMPTION AND
YOUR PERCEPTION
OF PRESSURE AND
URGENCY?

No!', regardless of whether the adrenaline that's there is the result of your overwhelming to-do list or an actual threat. A highly restricted diet with inadequate total food intake in combination with excessive exercise is another scenario that can communicate to your hypothalamus that you aren't safe. Your body doesn't know the difference between you eating very little due to a food shortage versus a conscious decision to 'go on a diet'.

So as soon as the 'I'm not safe' information is received by the hypothalamus (immediately, rapidly; faster than you can think), it sends this alert to the pituitary who immediately responds with her cascade of hormones to the other endocrine glands based on the 'no'. This is one reason why people who feel like their health is crashing, and start researching it, can't work out if they need to focus on the adrenals, the thyroid or their reproductive system, as all glands seem to be conveying symptoms that they are functioning sub-optimally (not diseased, just not working as well as they could be).

THEY WILL ALL HAVE BEEN ON THE RECEIVING END OF THE MESSAGE 'I'M NOT SAFE' ON REPEAT FOR YEARS OR EVEN DECADES.

How many days do you spend with elevated adrenaline due to your caffeine consumption and your perception of pressure and urgency? Really think about that and, consequently, how often your endocrine system is flooded with the message that you aren't safe.

EMOTIONALLY

Every human has a set of rules that they don't know about unless they've gone looking for what has to happen for them to feel a certain way—including to feel safe. When I've done this exercise with clients, when I ask them what has to happen for them to feel safe, the responses often cover a broad range of different areas of life. For example, for some people the first life department they reference when asked this question is about physical safety. They'll say they feel safe as long as the doors and windows are locked.

Others start talking to me about their finances—they feel like they need a certain amount of money in the bank or invested to feel safe, so they know that their future is taken care of in this way. Other people go straight to explaining how their relationships must be, particularly their intimate relationship or those with their inner circle.

They might say that they don't feel safe if they are on the receiving end of a raised voice on a regular basis. Other people tell me what has to be happening for their children if they are to feel safe. My point is, what is required for people to feel safe on an emotional level is highly varied. Yet if you have never explored this, chances are you live too many moments of too many days where the hypothalamus receives the message 'no' when it enquires if you are safe, due to your subconscious safety 'rules' not being met.

It is a worthwhile exercise to do. I suggest you do it now.

WHAT HAS TO HAPPEN FOR YOU TO FEEL SAFE?

Be sure to answer this for yourself. It is important you understand your own rules.

Here are some common ones that may resonate for you or prompt your own thinking and exploration of this concept.

I feel safe only if:

- My home is secure and I check the locks a few times before bed or going out.

- I feel like my skin is flawless, otherwise I feel like people will judge me or won't like me.

- My bank account has more than a certain level of money in it.

- My relationships with EVERYONE are peaceful and there is no conflict or tension.

- My children are getting excellent grades.

Your turn. What has to happen for you to feel safe?

After you do that, you may like to flip the question to ask and explore: What can never happen for you to feel safe?

Here are some examples to help you to start exploring this for yourself:

- He can never raise his voice at me.

- My best friend has to text me back really quickly otherwise I worry I've done something wrong or offended her somehow.

- If I send someone an email at work and don't hear back from them that day, I worry I've lost that customer or that they aren't happy with me; either way I worry this means we'll lose money.

After doing these exercises, it might be wise for you to write new rules about what has to happen for you to feel safe. Think of them like a blueprint (explored in this section on page 130). And work towards spending less time with your endocrine system spreading the message that you aren't safe, when indeed you are safe. You want to help your endocrine and nervous systems to foster more trust and less fear.

As humans we have a need to feel that who we are is enough, for our greatest fear, and hence where the greatest stress comes from, is that if we aren't enough then we won't be loved.

Reflect

WHAT HAS TO HAPPEN FOR YOU TO FEEL SAFE?

_____

_____

_____

_____

_____

_____

_____

_____

_____

_____

WHAT CAN NEVER HAPPEN FOR YOU TO FEEL SAFE?

_____

_____

_____

_____

_____

_____

_____

_____

_____

_____

_____

_____

What is common to all people is the emotional need for love and connection. But consider that this doesn't have to be with another person. It can be a faith, or a pet, or nature, or a divine love and appreciation for your own soul.

AS HUMANS WE HAVE A NEED TO FEEL THAT WHO WE ARE IS ENOUGH, FOR OUR GREATEST FEAR, AND HENCE WHERE THE GREATEST STRESS COMES FROM, IS THAT IF WE AREN'T ENOUGH THEN WE WON'T BE LOVED.

So foster that. You will never control how anyone else behaves towards you or responds to you or what they think of you. All of these things are usually a reflection of them, not you. So set up your rules of what has to happen to be safe as ones you are in charge of, rather than dependent on someone else to fulfil.

The goal with all of this—the physical and the emotional—is for the hypothalamus to be able to spread the message far more frequently throughout your whole body that you are safe. Your inner health and outer sparkle will love you for it ■

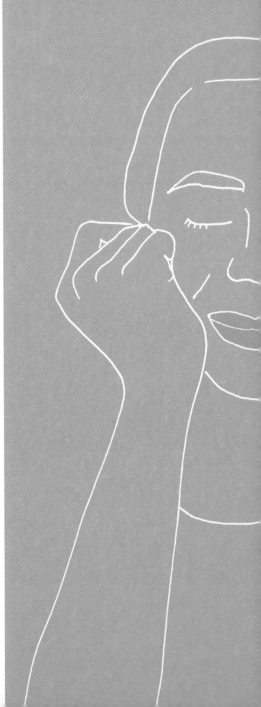

Dr Libby Weaver

> *She learned to stop*
> *walking out on herself.*
> *To stop letting herself down.*
> *So she stayed when it got hard.*
> *She believed in her*
> *own capacity to rise.*
> *And she saw it happen.*
> *And vowed to never stop*
> *believing in herself again.*

— Dr Rebecca Ray

When things aren't what you want them to be

Inner conflict

———

Given the impact that being perpetually stressed has on the speed at which we age, let's explore another way to minimise how much time you spend in that state. As humans, we have an overarching desire or expectation—consciously or subconsciously—about how our life is supposed to be. For some this is age-related: 'By the time I'm twenty-seven I need to be in a serious relationship and have an investment property.' For others, it is more general: 'My children need to be happy, healthy and doing well at school, and my work needs to be fulfilling but not too taxing on my time or energy.' This is what I'm going to refer to as your 'blueprint'. We can (unknowingly) create these blueprints from quite a young age when we imagine what our adult life is going to be like and we don't always realise they're there.

But if you have a blueprint of what life 'should' look like, and all the parts of your life aren't humming, or living up to how you pictured it to be, a sadness, deep stress, downtrodden lethargy or recurring anxious feelings might creep in. Often without us really being able to articulate why.

So, any friction between these known or unknown preconceived ideas about how life will look by a certain age (our blueprint), and/or how it is every day (our life conditions) can be a source of stress. We have a tendency to clump all the departments of life together and feel glum or joyous about their overall vibe. Yet, if you pause to reflect on each area your life, sure there may be a couple that aren't so flash (temporarily or long term) but the rest might be quite okay, or even rather wonderful.

LET'S DIG A LITTLE DEEPER ON THIS.

Work out what you consider to be your life departments (2). One might be your vitality, your health, your physical capacities. Another might be your vocation, career or occupation. The third might be your financial situation. The next, your relationships—your intimate relationship, friendships, relationships with colleagues, your children, your parents, your neighbours.

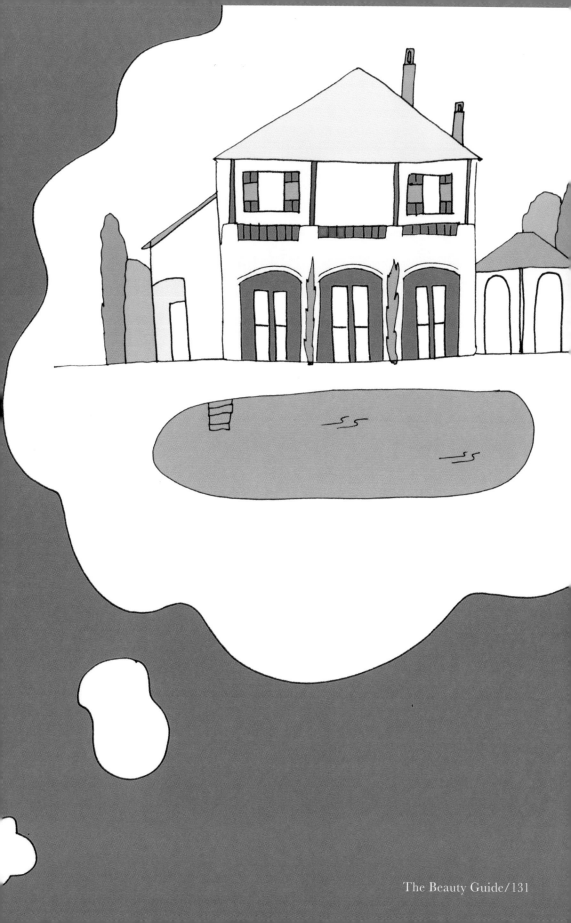

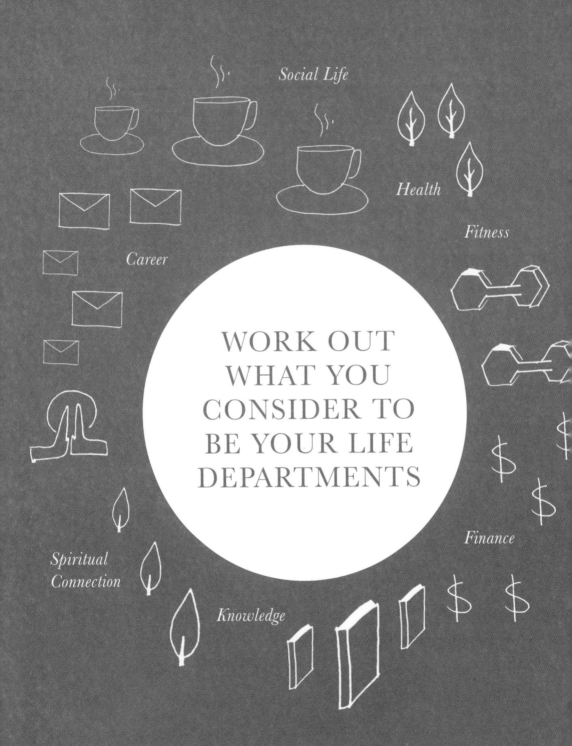

Social Life

Health

Fitness

Career

WORK OUT
WHAT YOU
CONSIDER TO
BE YOUR LIFE
DEPARTMENTS

Finance

Spiritual
Connection

Knowledge

Dr Libby Weaver

nother life department might be your spiritual connection, whether that be faith, with Nature or the Universe; you feel connected to and a part of something beyond yourself.

Perhaps a quest for knowledge, mental stimulation, growth and learning another life department for you. You continually seek to understand more about the world and love nothing more than a deep dive into a topic.

And yet another one might be your social interaction, or social leadership; reflective of how people respond to what we have to share. You might even see social leadership as parenting if you have children and cross-correlate this department with your relationships area.

WHEN YOU FEEL DOWN OR ANXIOUS OR STRESSED OUT, IT CAN BE BECAUSE YOU PERCEIVE THAT HOW LIFE IS RIGHT NOW IS NOT MATCHING UP WITH HOW YOU THINK IT IS SUPPOSED TO BE.

You're comparing your blueprint to your current conditions and feeling that something is lacking. Yet in the seven areas, there might only be two where you're not satisfied, while the other five are in a good place. We tend to place too much emphasis on one or two of the bucket/s—often the ones that aren't how we want them to be (it's the black dot on the white paper story in action; refer to page 160)—and we think that one will mess up our whole life. That's how stress can feel like it is permeating your entire existence and begin to overwhelm you.

Is it even possible for all of your life departments to be where you want them to be all the time? No way. You'd never grow if that was the case; we typically learn and grow from our challenges rather than our joys. One way to look at it is that, if you're not winning, you're growing.

So, if we recognise that our life conditions versus our blueprint is a major factor (or even just a contributing factor) in our stress or sadness or downtrodden lethargy or anxious feelings, what can we do about it? You can alter one or the other.

There are times when we can change our life conditions and times when we can't. You might want to quit your job, for example, but doing so immediately would bring more stress with the ripple effect it would create… at the moment. Or perhaps you may decide to start your own business and just need more time for that to become more financially prosperous before quitting your day job. In time, you may be presented with another opportunity in a field you are more passionate about or maybe your financial situation changes and you're able to focus on growing your business. So one option is to change your life conditions.

The other, changing your blueprint, can be just as effective—although some find this harder. Here's an example I witnessed in a colleague recently…

In parts of New Zealand and Australia, we have been living for a while in what real estate people refer to as a property boom, or a bubble. In other words, house prices are exorbitantly high, particularly in major cities.

In *Rushing Woman's Syndrome*, I made a statement that 'no house is worth it'. I wanted people to reflect on what their mortgage was costing them in terms of their life quality and their health. It was also in response to what I'd heard hundreds, if not thousands, of women intimate. There is no doubt that many women work because they love it, yet there are also those who work in jobs that don't inspire them only to pay the mortgage (their partners work as well in the cases I'm referring to). And they are stretched; often self-reportedly beyond their limits and, really, against their will and self-care knowledge—trying to juggle work, the needs of their families and the financial demands of their life. Their blueprint might be that to be 'successful' they need to own a four-bedroom house

in a nice neighbourhood, close to a good school in a major city. Let's say this house will cost them $2 million. Yet if they change their blueprint and relish relocating to a smaller city or town, they might obtain those same criteria for $750,000. This is often prompted by pondering the question: what does being debt free offer you?

Instead of living on credit card debt, working two jobs, always tired, and rarely seeing your children, changing your blueprint about what life is suppose to look like could lead you to create a completely different way of life.

IS IT EVEN POSSIBLE FOR ALL OF YOUR LIFE DEPARTMENTS TO BE WHERE YOU WANT THEM TO BE ALL THE TIME? NO WAY.

As I mentioned earlier, instead of trying to work out how to make ends meet, another option is to work on having fewe ends (1). I know this example of moving from the city to the country and buying a cheaper house doesn't suit everyone. I'm simply sharing what occurred for a colleague and the insights I caught a glimpse of while she was sharing with me the health benefits all of this brought her

Another example is from a delightful patient of mine from a few years ago. Her definition of success very much revolved around how she looked, particularly her clothes. It was essential, yes essential, for her to have four to six brand-new tailor-made suits every year, even though there was nothing wrong with the ones from the year before. To go with her new suits, each year she'd buy at least 20 new business shirts and she wore ties—she owned hundreds of them. She said she felt like a failure if she didn't pull all of this off: the beautiful suits, shirts, ties and shoes. She'd started to get weary of her line of work though, and didn't feel fulfilled by her job any more.

On top of this, her energy was through the floor and her skin had started to break out in her forties, which distressed her. She didn't know how she could ever change her life to regain her health as she was sure she'd feel like a failure every minute of every day if she didn't hit her fashion targets. I knew she wouldn't change her life conditions (although sometimes this is forced on us via health challenges) and because I knew her family history, I understood where this 'need' stemmed from, so I suggested she start exploring the blueprints of her life buckets. Like everything, she embraced this with gusto.

Over the following year, her new measure of success grew to be about being able to get dressed in less than five minutes. She now feels happy, successful (a word that is still important to her) and juiced about life wearing shorts and a T-shirt each day. She certainly overhauled her blueprint and has reaped the rewards of less stress, more joy and better health and energy. Plus, her skin cleared up. This case study might be an extreme example, but I share it to show you that anything is possible.

So, if you feel like the stress in your life stems from an unrelenting dissatisfaction, I hope exploring your life conditions and your blueprint, and possibly combining this work with that described in the 'Am I Safe?' section (refer to page 122), brings you the beauty, inner peace and grace that a life lived in congruence with your true values offers you ■

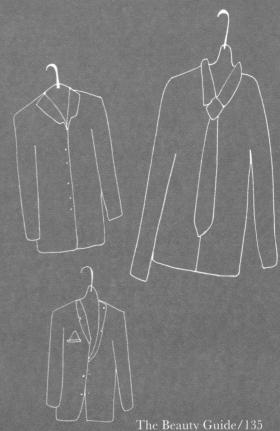

EXERCISE

Take some time now to get honest with yourself, to reflect on your own life conditions and blueprint and some steps you might be able to take to get these more in alignment.

First you may like to identify your life departments. If it helps, use the ones in this chapter to prompt you.

Then, start in the left-hand column: the 'Blueprint'. If you are truly honest, what vision did or do you hold for your life? What do you dream about having, being or doing?

Now move to the right-hand column: 'Life Conditions'. What is your life like right now? In comparison to the things you wrote down in the Blueprint column? Do these look like the lives of two separate people or are there some commonalities between them?

Now look at the middle column: 'Changes you can make'. Reflecting on the 'Blueprint' column, what are some steps you could take to offer more congruency between these two columns? It might be adjusting your current life conditions or reconsidering your blueprint. It might be big steps or just smaller, more everyday changes that you can take ■

LIFE DEPARTMENTS

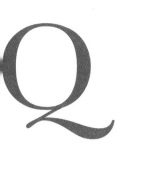

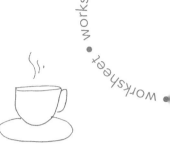

Q

BLUEPRINT	CHANGES YOU CAN MAKE	LIFE CONDITIONS

Lifting the veil on your values

What do you truly care about?

Knowing who you are and being true to that is one of the most important paths of learning you will ever take. Living out of alignment with your values does not promote a relaxed facial expression, upright posture, graceful movements, great energy or exceptional health. It does the opposite. It creates a deep tension that no amount of breathing or magnesium can alleviate.

One of the most important exercises you will ever do as far as living a life of integrity with yourself, and therefore generating less stress and subsequent regeneration, is one that helps you discover what your values are. I personally very much appreciate Dr John Demartini's work in this area. This includes his live events and book, *The Values Factor* (1), as well as his definition of values and the way he teaches you to discover yours.

Dr Demartini proposes that many of our values emerge from, and are subsequently determined by, our conscious or unconscious voids (2). What he means by this is, what you value deeply tends to arise from the things you perceive as most missing from your life or from within yourself (2). For example, you might see a successful businessperson and then discover they had an upbringing where money was very tight. So, as an adult, they have a high value around making money, which is ultimately driven by the void created by growing up in a household that was always worried about where the next dollar was coming from.

It may be of no surprise to you that my highest value is health. When I trace this back, in my early twenties I had an experience where my level of health went significantly south. In other words, I caught a glimpse of what life could be like not living with great health. In this state, my perceived lack of health created a void, which forged my highest value of health and a desire to share that with the world so that others did not have to suffer.

Dr Demartini explains that your values drive what you think about and your actions, and the bigger the void, the more importance you place on the value. For example, you may have been told as a young person, by someone you looked up to, that you are stupid and will never amount to anything. If you believed them and took on the belief that you are stupid (the void), you might value intelligence, learning, and expressing yourself in an erudite way.

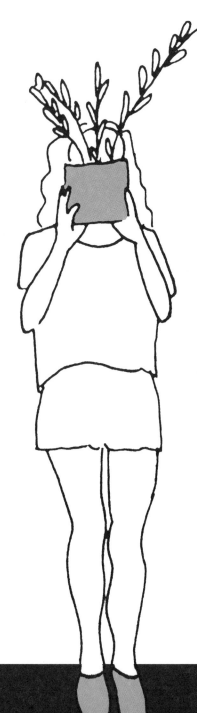

"
And if I asked you to
NAME ALL
OF THE
THINGS
YOU LOVE,
*how long would it take
for you to name yourself?*
"

– Anonymous

Dr Libby Weaver

Or that void might create an adult who values 'winning' or 'success' and who goes on to create a coaching business to help others be successful. Another example might be that while you were growing up, boys liked your friends and not you. Unknowingly, you created a belief that you weren't attractive (the void). As an adult, you do all you can to present yourself to the world in an 'attractive' way, never being seen without makeup on, your hair done and wearing the latest fashion trends. You value looking good.

Your values (and your voids) create a huge part of your life. They can impact significantly on the unfolding of your life and the choices you make, from the biggest to the smallest. Think jobs, partners, whether you have children or not, whether you buy organic produce, throw food out or use up every last morsel.

A fulfilling life and the ability to appreciate yourself enough to take excellent care of your health involves filling your perceptually empty voids. Because, unless we recognise that they are there, our voids will operate behind the scenes without us realising it, often fostering disharmony or inner conflict.

For example, you might *think* you want great health, but unconsciously you don't place a high value around it, and so shopping, cooking or making food for yourself feels like too much to bother with. Until you move health higher up your values, you will typically seek external 'motivation' to help you find 'inspiration' to provide yourself with more nutritious food more regularly. You want someone else to tell you what to do yet you can't sustain their guidance. For when we aren't inwardly motivated to take the best care of ourselves, it will be something that easily slips, and you might find yourself in a seesaw between getting healthy and falling back into old habits of relying on takeout and eating whatever is quickest and easiest. This is the result of consciously knowing that you need to take care of yourself (we aren't impervious to the messages we hear about nutrition and exercise) but not having health as a highly valued priority.

THE CONFLICT BETWEEN YOUR CONSCIOUS AND UNCONSCIOUS VALUES IS LIKELY TO BRING YOU STRESS IN MORE THAN ONE WAY.

You have the stress to your body of not providing it with adequate antioxidants and nutrients, as well as the stress of worrying that you aren't doing a good enough job in this area—the ultimate stress (or what I prefer to call fear, explored on page 111).

So with all of this in mind, let's begin to work out what your values are and create the possibility for you to live more aligned with them—with all of the health and beauty benefits that brings.

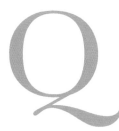

All values explorations ask you to honestly look at what your life demonstrates as being truly important to you. After all, we make time for what we prioritise. It is entirel understandable if you initially don't know what your answers are. You may find yourse wanting to answer inaccurately, wistfully describing how you wish your life was, or in ways that you think are socially acceptable, for example ■

1 STEP ONE

Consider what you fill your space with. What is around you? Name three things For me, there are always books in my environments, no matter where I am—at home, in the office, in my luggage or beside my bed (even in a hotel room).

1. _____

2. _____

3. _____

2 STEP TWO

Consider carefully how you spend your time. What are the three things that you spend your time on most? For most adults it is 'work'; however, be specific about what you do. Do you spend most of your time 'communicating' or 'driving' or 'researching' or 'helping people' as part of your work day? Be specific.

1. _____

2. _____

3. _____

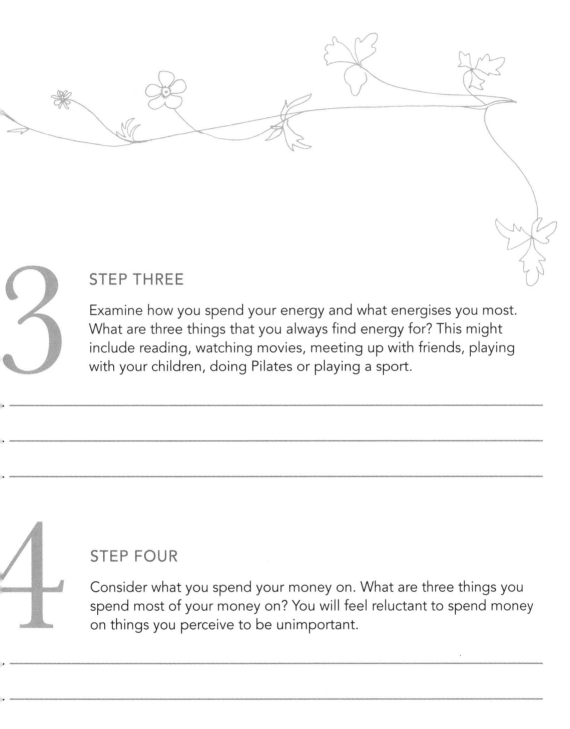

3 STEP THREE

Examine how you spend your energy and what energises you most. What are three things that you always find energy for? This might include reading, watching movies, meeting up with friends, playing with your children, doing Pilates or playing a sport.

_____

_____

_____

4 STEP FOUR

Consider what you spend your money on. What are three things you spend most of your money on? You will feel reluctant to spend money on things you perceive to be unimportant.

_____

_____

_____

5

STEP FIVE

Look for repetition; you may be expressing something using different language, but the value will be the same. For example, for me, many of my answers included things like organic food, organic skincare, tennis, Pilates, nature—for me this is all health, my version of holistic health so I group them all together. Group similar answers together until you have a few different categories. Then name those categories.

Reflect

What came out at number one? This is the category with the most answers in it.

Were you surprised? Or delighted? Is this how you want life to be?

Or is there something you can now see needs to change?

For example, perhaps you spend most of your time and energy working (during work hours as well as after hours) and maybe this isn't what you'd like to see in your number one spot. Maybe you'd like to spend more time and energy with your children and/or cultivating a stronger relationship with your partner or ageing parents.

Now think about what you learnt earlier about the way stress compromises the non-essential processes, i.e. the beauty bits. You might want your hair or skin or nails to look a certain way, but are your current values supporting or standing in the way of you experiencing this?

My goal in suggesting you examine this is to help bring more peace and less conflict and struggle to your life and perceptions, as well as the perceptions of the body. Harmony is a catalyst to beauty, both in your expression of the light in your heart as well as your appreciation of the beauty in your world.

Remember, you lack nothing—it is just a perception. Yet these perceptions of our voids contribute to creating our values and therefore what we act on. This can also serve the world as our voids are usually what drive us to contribute—and there is immense beauty in contribution.

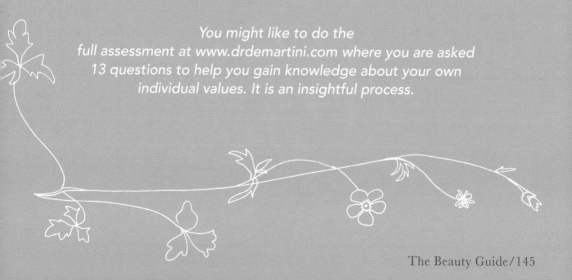

*You might like to do the
full assessment at www.drdemartini.com where you are asked
13 questions to help you gain knowledge about your own
individual values. It is an insightful process.*

Create more calm

Tips to de-stress

How can you decrease your stress response? The intensity of it, as well as how much time you spend in this place? Given that the relentless output of stress hormones is strongly linked to a host of health challenges, including those that are visible on the outside, how can you communicate more frequently to your body that i is safe? Here are some suggestions.

1 Consume less caffeine from all sources, as caffeine blocks the adenosine receptors in the brain and activates the stress axis, sending a signal to the adrenals to make adrenaline.

2 Increase your intake of antioxidants from whole, real plant foods with a wide variety of colours. You need the oxygen donation these foods offer to mop up th free radicals that are generated when yo breathe more rapidly, which occurs wher adrenaline is elevated.

3 Ensure you are obtaining optimal levels of B vitamins, vitamin C and magnesium. A wide variety of whole, real foods contain B vitamins, although foods derived from animals are the only ones that contain vitamin B12. Vitamin C is found in citrus fruits, kiwifruit and capsicum, while magnesium is found predominantly in green leafy vegetables, nuts and seeds. Remember that the more units of stress hormones you produce, the greater your requirement for these nutrients.

4 Explore your perception of pressure and urgency and save it for when you really need it. For example, if you get a phone call from your child's school and learn that they have been injured, it is urgent for you to get to the school. If a car pulls out in front of you, it is urgent for you to slam on your brakes. If you receive 300 new emails overnight, you will likely feel that all of them are urgent in your overwhelmed and/or caffeinated (promoting elevated adrenaline already) state, when in reality maybe 10 need your attention quit quickly. Although, in the latter example no life is in danger so on a scale of urgency, this is lower than the first two, just to point out the obvious.

5 When you look at your to-do list, remember how privileged your life is because all your basic needs are met and still for too many people in the world, this is not the case. It can help to remember that you 'get' to do all of this, rather than you 'have' to. We are, after all, busy with what we say yes to.

6 Cultivate better energy (refer to page 33), for when you have great energy, your choices and thoughts are more conducive to seeing things as they are—not worse than they are, or better than they are, just as they are. This helps us to stay calm.

7 Diaphragmatically breathe: this activates the calm arm of the nervous system (the parasympathetic nervous system), to become breath aware. Embrace a breath-focused practice or establish rituals in your day so that you regularly do long, slow breaths.

8 Explore whether your body has been getting the message that you aren't safe through physical or emotional stimuli by completing the reflection on page 127.

9 Examine whether what is referred to as your 'Life Conditions' (LC) equal your 'Blueprint' (BP) (1). In other words, does how it is (LC) match up to how you think it is supposed to be (BP). I have even heard it argued in some pioneering medical circles that feeling down is essentially the result of our LC not equalling our BP (explored on page 130).

10 If you feel that stress is really at the heart of your beauty challenges, then I urge you to consider this. The real word for stress is fear. Whatever you are stressed about—anything at all—is usually what you are frightened of. Peel back the layers on what you perceive are your stresses—running late, for example—and see what's really there. See what you are actually afraid of. Of being a failure, of being seen as lazy, of people not liking you, of letting others down... For most people, when they peel it all back, their fear is that they are not loved, or that there will be a loss of love. Everything—and I mean everything—comes back to avoiding rejection and obtaining or maintaining love. I don't know how else to say it. People think the opposite of stressed is relaxed or calm. I say it is trust ■

SELF.

image

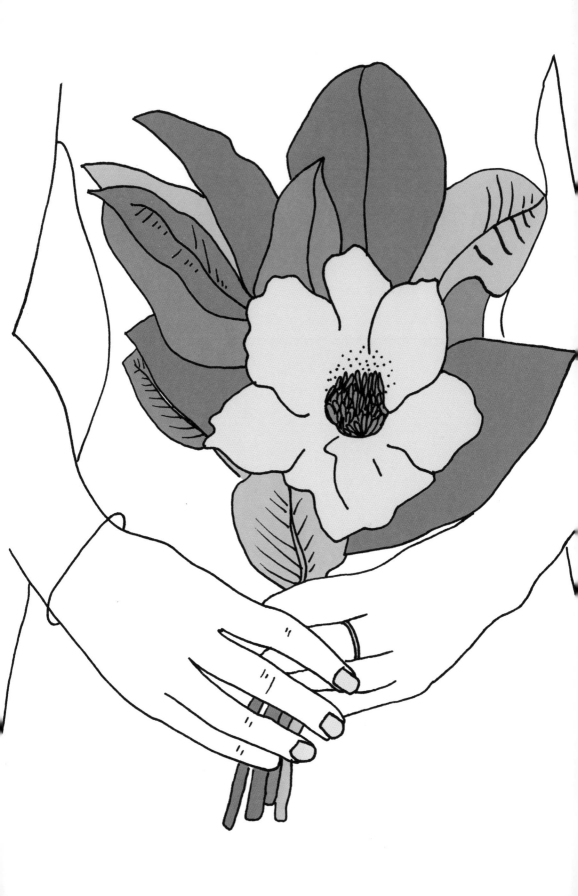

Caring is beautiful

The origin of true beauty

Whatever you touch, do it with care. Whether it is your face, your arms, university or work project, or someone else's heart, bring your attention to the concept of caring and act from that place. Sometimes caring has a tender and gentle tone of voice. However, at other times, caring involves intensity.

For example, if a child has run out into the road and a car is coming, the caring way to act is to alert the child to impending danger. But the intention behind this intense way of speaking and acting comes from a place of deep caring. Yet if you'd left a message for or texted a friend and you hadn't heard back for a while, and you are fretting that you've offended her or that she doesn't like you any more… and then when she contacts you, you yell at her, is that from caring or from fear? It's from fear. The scenario scratched the itch of your 'not enoughness'. Yet if you enquired if she was okay (caring), and simply expressed that you were worried, she will likely share with you that she's been overwhelmed with tasks and missing you and looking forward to the next time you catch up.

Speaking intensely with care is quite different to speaking from a place of judgement. When you judge another person, it is a reflection of your own pain—it says nothing about them—and doesn't demonstrate care for yourself or the other. If you notice yourself judging someone, bring curiosity to the situation so you can gain insights about why you feel you might be judging them. You might run into an old flame (who broke your heart) with their new partner and immediately find yourself making judgements about the type of person their new partner might be. Bring compassion to yourself, as we judge from places where we don't feel like we are enough, in moments when we have forgotten to live from the truth of who we are… which is love. Or in this situation, if you notice many of your judgements stem from heartbreak, you could recall the words of the poet Rudy Francisco who said: (1)

> *"INSTEAD OF ASKING WHY THEY LEFT, NOW I ASK WHAT BEAUTY WILL I CREATE IN THE SPACE THEY NO LONGER OCCUPY?"*

" *If you're pretty,
you're pretty.*
BUT THE ONLY
WAY TO BE
BEAUTIFUL IS
TO BE CARING
AND LOVING.

Otherwise, it's just

'Congratulations about your face.'

"

– Anonymous

One of my concerns in this age of rapidly advancing technology is that too many people may be losing touch with the importance of care and consideration in certain settings. Would you actually say those words you wrote aloud if the person were standing in front of you? If you elevated caring on your values list, would you even phrase it that way in the first place? Pause before you post, write or say something, and reflect on whether you are touching the situation with care.

There is so much beauty in caring—about others, about the planet, and about the wellbeing of your own body, mind and soul.

You can actively choose to bring caring to the forefront of your values, your thoughts, your actions and your beauty routine.

List what you will 'touch' with more care ▨

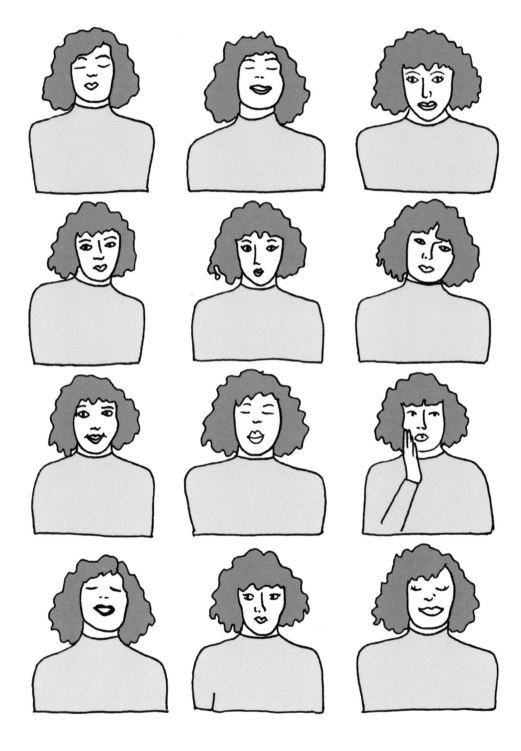

Culture of comparison

Measuring your reality against someone else's highlight reel

When you see photos of people you don't know—i.e. who you can't see in real life—on social media, how are you supposed to know what is real and what is filtered, airbrushed or digitally altered. What happens to our own minds when we constantly see faces that we think are 'beautiful' in the traditional meaning of the word, without any real knowledge of whether it accurately reflects how they look like in real life or the way they were born? The number of women seeking cosmetic treatments and surgery is growing, and it's not just older women trying to counteract the signs of ageing—women as young as eighteen are getting Botox as a 'preventative' measure.

When we look at an image of someone, we don't always know if something has been plumped up from injections, surgically adjusted or tattooed to look fuller and more defined. And while, on the one hand, it's wonderful that we have avenues through which to make ourselves feel better about our appearance, I also believe we need to be more transparent and ensure that younger people (and older ones for that matter) are acutely aware that what they are seeing may not be attainable in nature. Because too many younger girls don't understand the difference. Too many of the ones I speak to believe what they see, and ingrained in them is a belief that they are failing or ugly or not good enough if they don't match up to what they see.

What tends to happen in our minds, when we see a similar style of image over and over again, is we start to think that is what 'normal' looks like; that what we're exposed to through advertising and social media is how we are all supposed to look. We compare ourselves to what we see and if we don't look like that, our mind might tell us that there is something wrong with us and that there are (many) things we need to change. It is the not enoughness that I talk about in all my work, on another scale.

When I was growing up, some girls had Barbie dolls and I remember being taught that her shape was unattainable—the ratio of her bust to waist to hips was not possible in nature. But she was just a doll. Now there are non-stop images available to young (and mature) women who, if they aren't in touch with their own enoughness, are prepared to risk their health to have themselves artificially altered or constructed because they perceive that what they were born with is not enough.

When it comes to the long-term effects of these choices, we truly are in the dark. When substances are tested for safety, they're not tested over a long period of time or to assess how our body might respond if we continue to top up on a regular basis. The illnesses that can occur due to breast implants are now rife, for example. How are you to know that what is deemed 'safe' today won't be banned in years to come because of the detrimental toxic load or immune system challenges that can arise from having chemicals injected or foreign objects put inside you? While there are many substances that may be safe and not create problematic issues further down the track, there have been numerous occasions since the inception of breast implants where products used were deemed unsuitable for future use due to thousands of women getting sick. There are now online groups created to support women experiencing the immense distress of these sicknesses—which they often don't initially recognise for what they are and spend years perplexed about why they feel so unwell.

_____

NEVER BEFORE HAVE WE HAD SO MANY FOREIGN OBJECTS ON OFFER TO PUT INTO OUR BODIES.

_____

We have no idea of the short or long-term consequences of their use as they haven't been around long enough for us to know them all yet.

Please don't get me wrong. None of this is to say that altering your appearance or opting for cosmetic procedures is wrong or a negative thing. I can remember the first person I knew who yearned to save enough money for a facelift and while she was under the anaesthetic, she was going to have the extra skin removed from between her eyes and her eyebrows. She was incredibly self-conscious of this at age 62. At this stage in her life, she'd very sadly nursed two husbands to their death and all she saw when she looked at her own face was the sadness of her past. I had such empathy for her and completely understood why this surgery was so important to her. I have immense empathy for younger women too, who feel that surgery is the only way. Yet I don't want their choices to be made from a belief in their own deficiency. It is so important that you come to know what is motivating your decisions. And all I want is for your decision to stem from love, not fear.

It pains me that too many women fear the changes in their body—they fear people will think differently of them if they aren't young or beautiful in the traditional context of the word. And it is this fear as the driving force behind someone seeking cosmetic changes that I am speaking about here, not the cosmetic surgery itself.

Yet, as you now understand, our voids contribute to creating our values and, even if we do operate from this place of fear, there is still an opportunity for growth for us. So, if you believe that you aren't pretty enough, hot enough, desirable enough or beautiful enough, the journey you undertake to fill your perceived void will lead you to experience things that you may not have done without that void. And for many people, this void, and the consequent experiences, leads us to contribute further down the track. And I trust completely in the unfolding of that.

Pema Chodron, the wonderful Buddhist teacher, says it beautifully when she says:

Our life's work is to use what we have been given to wake up. If there were two people who were exactly the same—same body, same speech, same mind, same mother, same father, same house, same food, everything the same—one of them could use what he has to wake up and the other could use it to become more resentful, bitter, and sour. It doesn't matter what you're given, whether it's physical deformity or enormous wealth or poverty, beauty or ugliness, mental stability or mental instability, life in the middle of a madhouse or life in the middle of a peaceful, silent desert. Whatever you're given can wake you up or put you to sleep."(1)

These beautiful words lead me to my other concern: what we miss when we plaster over something that has potentially appeared to help wake us up. For if a new line has appeared, let's say somewhere on your face, it can indicate that an inner organ needs support, or that there is a nutritional deficiency or that you've had a repeated facial expression and behind that expression is an emotion, the basis of which needs to be understood so that you learn and grow. If you get rid of the irritant (the new wrinkle), you can miss the message, as you won't be focused on deciphering what the message may be. For you to believe that a wrinkle has appeared as a gift to you, you have to believe that life happens for you, not to you. When you inject it away, you can miss the message.

That's the challenge of now: what are you going to do with what you have already—your body, your speech, your mind? The things that you find challenging and the things that you love. For every moment, we get to choose what we focus on and choose how our perceived voids shape our experience of life.

So, the real question is: do you feel the desire, the need or the longing to live in a different way? To not get caught up in the trappings of a perceived 'not enoughness' and all of the ways that can play out. To live with ease and spaciousness, energy and vitality, your inner light beaming out from within, exactly as you are. To make different choices if you have been acting from this place of fear. To stop punishing yourself or shaming yourself or telling yourself that you are a failure and not okay the way you are.

THE PUNISHMENT OF YOURSELF HAS TO STOP.

Not only in your judgements of your own appearance, your relationship with food and lifestyle choices, but in your relationships with other people, with work, with money, and, most importantly, with yourself. And if you do stop, that gives you a choice about what to do, how to eat, what you put your attention on, what your priorities are, how you perceive yourself and how you live. And it is your way of life that this book is about—a way to gently, nurturingly, with ease and grace, love and support what nature has so graciously given you.

My intention with this book is to help you live a life with a reservoir and a daily experience of a deep appreciation for yourself. A self-love that allows you to experience all that is on offer to you, and allows you to share your gifts. Because regardless of how you look, your age or the body into which you have been born, you have so many gifts to offer the world, exactly as you are ∎

Dr Libby Weaver

> " EMBRACE YOUR INDIVIDUALITY
>
> # LOVE WHAT YOU LOVE
>
> WITHOUT WORRYING ABOUT JUDGEMENT.
> "
>
> — *Anonymous*

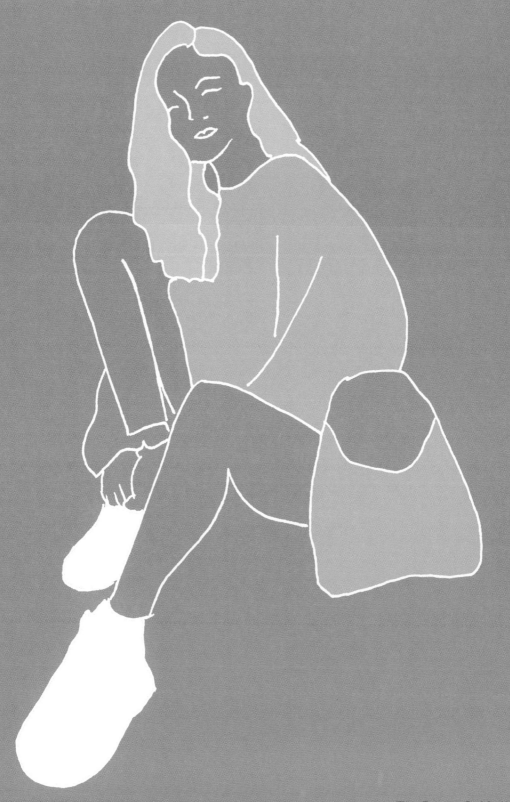

Laser focus

What are you not seeing?

An experiment went around the traps a few years ago. The story goes something like this…

A teacher announced to her classroom that they were going to have an unexpected test.

The students waited anxiously to find out what it was about.

The teacher handed out the paper and placed it face down on the desk, in the way all their tests are placed.

When she asked them to turn it over, the only thing on the page was a small black dot in the centre of the page.

The task at hand—the test—was for the students to simply write about what they saw.

At the conclusion of the test period, the students handed in their papers.

Every single one of them, with no exceptions, wrote about the black dot. About its position on the page, its colour, its size. Not one single student wrote about the white part of the paper. Everyone focused on the black dot. It was as if they didn't even see the white paper.

And that's what we do with our lives. We focus on our equivalent of the black dot. Challenges or disappointments with friends or colleagues, financial concerns, relationship complications, the size of our body or a particular body part…

Yet the black dots in our lives are very small compared to everything else we have in our lives. Why is it that this is what most people choose to focus on?

This just creates a vicious cycle of poor-quality thoughts as one tends to lead to another and another. In just the same way, 'white paper' (abundance, gratitude etc.) thoughts foster each other and the simple act of redirecting your focus to what you do have can make an incredible difference to the quality of your life.

SPEND FAR LESS TIME FOCUSING ON THE BLACK DOTS AND LIVE MORE IN TOUCH WITH THE GIFTS THAT EACH MOMENT OF LIFE OFFERS YOU.

And notice how different you feel inside and out ■

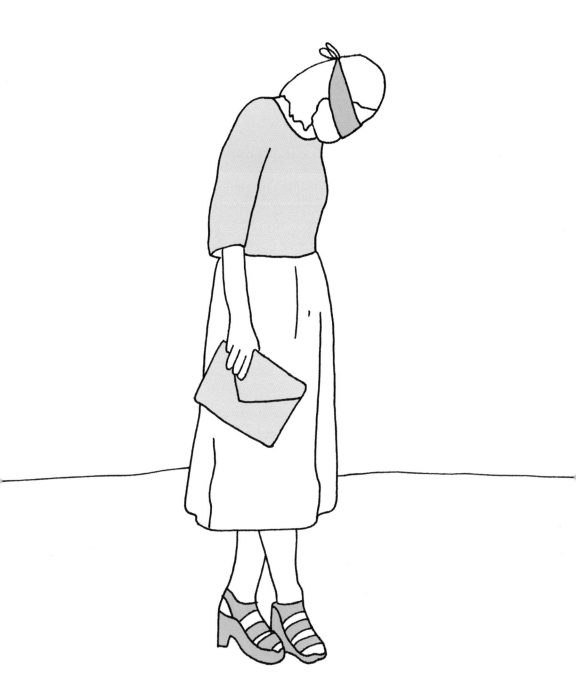

Your black dot

Write down, inside the circle on the opposite page, your biggest worry or frustration at the moment. This could be anything from what's going on in the world to your body, your family, your relationships or a particular relationship, or financial concerns. Just pick one worry and write it in the circle.

Then, in the space around the black circle, write everything that's good about that worry. All the things that you've actioned, changed or transformed because of that worry. Think of the things that may or may not have happened because of that worry. Get creative.

EXAMPLE:

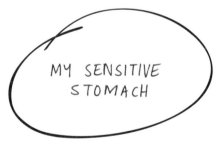

INTEREST IN
COOKING DELICIOUS
MEALS FOR
MYSELF

LEARNING
ABOUT DIGESTION

INCREASED
AWARENESS
ABOUT DIGESTION

LIVE MORE
IN TOUCH
WITH MY
EMOTIONS

MY SENSITIVE
STOMACH

CONNECTION WITH
MY HEALTH &
BODY

THINKING BEFORE
EATING IMPULSIVELY

FOUND YOGA

LESS WHEAT
& DAIRY WOULD
HAVE HELPED
OTHER AREAS
OF MY HEALTH

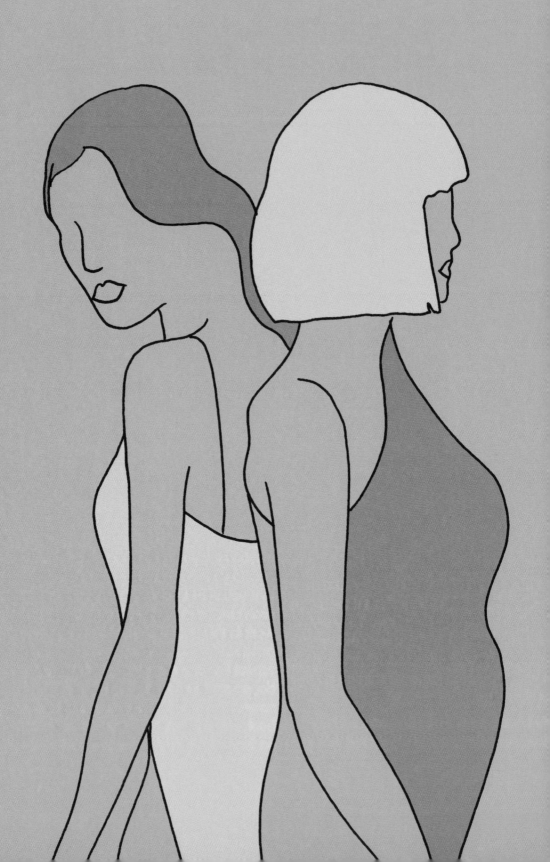

Weighing in on body fat

Is self-judgement dimming your light?

What is the first thing you think about when you think of beauty? Is it the glistening eyes of someone you think is wonderful? Is it the kindness that beams out of the actions of a person you appreciate? Does it involve skin being radiant or smooth in its texture? Or is it all about body fat and body tone?

Still today for too many women of all ages, concerns about body fat and image run their thinking, their life and their choices. Regardless of their size, it often involves a relentless stream of negotiations in their mind and is yet another way they scratch the itch of their not enoughness. And it can be some of the cruellest, most unsupportive inner dialogue you ever did hear. You'd ditch your friend if she spoke to you like this.

Not only does this harsh self-judgement drive us to dim our light and lead to the relentless output of stress hormones as well as other health-negating consequences, we can end up missing, not only all of the beauty that surrounds us, but the beauty within us and the beauty that we are.

When you talk to people who are dying and ask them what they are going to miss the most they tell you the most ordinary things. No one mentions that they'll miss living as the size they were, whatever that size was. In the end, whenever that is, you won't care about the size of your thighs or your waist, or how toned your shoulders look. So why wait until then to wake up?

I'm all for living a life that fosters great health and energy and, in my experience, when we are healthy, our body fat levels become what is best for us. We need body fat for countless reasons. We stop menstruating, for example, if we don't keep enough of it on our bones. It also helps our brain to think, produces hormones, keeps us warm and protects the organs that keep us alive—among many other tasks.

THERE IS ALSO NO ONE WAY FOR US ALL TO LOOK AS FAR AS BODY FAT LEVELS GO.

Shift your attention and intention to having great energy and a strong, functional, flexible body, rather than on body fat levels or your weight and see what unfolds. With a focus on the former, you live in a world of abundance. With a focus on the latter, it's all about deprivation and what you can't have—and no one can sustain that. Nor is it a healthy mindset. There is no question, however, that too little or too much body fat often comes along with some lousy health consequences. So, we can accept ourselves as we are, while still cultivating a life and lifestyle choices that may involve changing body fat levels (to be higher or lower) so that we have the right amount, for us, as individuals. Whatever that is.

You want muscles so that you can carry groceries and your grandchildren when you are eighty and still live independently.

You want the right amount of body fat for you so that you don't die too young of heart failure if it is too low or cardiovascular disease if it is too high.

Or you can make your body tone and musculature, your body fat levels and what you eat all about how you look. Whether you reveal this to anyone or not.

I cannot encourage you enough to embrace, accept and appreciate your body as it is right now. That doesn't have to mean that there may not be things you want to alter—the clarity of your skin or the size of your thighs—but please foster these changes through a focus on health, through a desire to care for yourself because you deeply appreciate your 'self and your gift of life. The weight-focused road is typically filled with suffering. The health and energy focused road offers you freedom.

And there is so much beauty in freedom.

YOU WANT TO EAT NUTRIENT-DENSE FOODS BECAUSE YOU WANT GREAT ENERGY.

Dr Libby Weaver

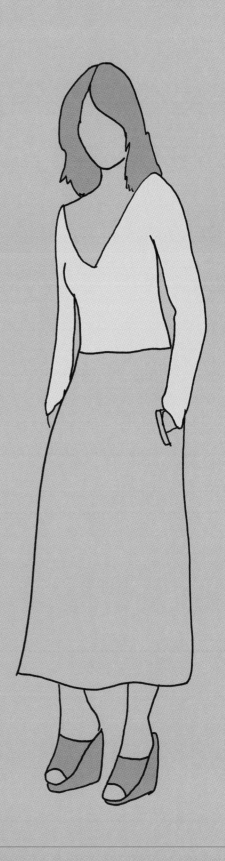

> "
>
> That's the thing about inner beauty: *unlike physical beauty, which grabs the spotlight for itself,*
>
> INNER BEAUTY SHINES ON EVERYONE, CATCHING THEM, HOLDING THEM IN ITS EMBRACE, MAKING THEM MORE BEAUTIFUL TOO.
>
> "
>
> – *Anonymous*

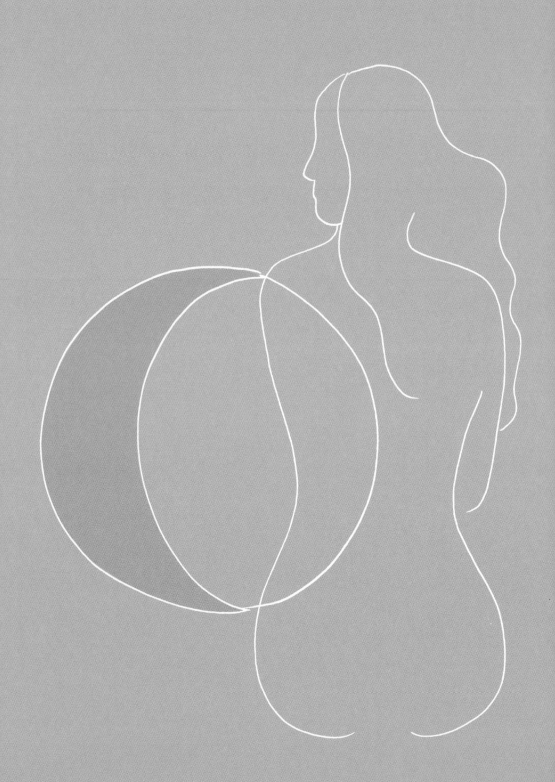

The miracle of your body

And living in touch with it

While living in a flat with friends through my years at uni, I had a pimple on my neck. One of my flatmates walked into the bathroom while I was giving it a good old squeeze. She told me not to squeeze it as it might scar. I must have said something derogatory about my neck and she said, 'You should be grateful you have a neck.' We laughed but her light-hearted statement hit me with a wallop of truth. How often do you put yourself down for something you don't like when you could so easily shift your focus to the fact that the particular body part functions and that you have been gifted with it in the first place? For example, 'I hate my cellulite' could become 'I'm so grateful my legs carry me everywhere I need to go'. By all means, you can learn about and take actions to decrease why you might have cellulite, but don't be miserable about it.

WHEN YOU FEEL GRATEFUL IT GIVES YOU FUEL—ENERGY—TO TAKE ACTION IN YOUR LIFE AND APPRECIATE YOURSELF.

If you catch yourself in self-judgement, flip it immediately into steps you can take to change what it is. Supporting your liver for clearer skin, for example, or changing your perception of it: 'It's here to teach me something. I don't yet know what that is, but I'll get the message when the time is right.'

A friend of mine who is in a wheelchair due to an accident has shared so much with me about this concept. She's done the New York and other marathons, including one in the Himalayas using a hand cycle (a bike you pedal with your hands). She was out training using a hand cycle on her local roads (she is well known in her local area and, in fact, nationally in her home country for her pioneering, champion spirit and achievements) when someone drove past and shouted out 'You are amazing!' When recounting the story to me she said that she appreciated the encouragement of course but her words were: 'I don't want to be amazing. I just want to walk again.' She's not worrying about what parts of her look like. She's taking care of her extraordinary body via the way she looks after herself while raising money for a charity to help find a cure for spinal cord damage, so she can dance with her husband again.

You have a body that allows you to get about and do what you want to do in a day. It is made up of about 50 trillion cells (a crazy large number) and coordinates billions of biochemical reactions that create how you look and feel every minute of every day—all without you having to tell it to do so. Every day, your heart beats about 100,000 times and pumps about 7,500 litres of blood through about 96,000 kilometres of blood vessels.

YOU ARE AN ABSOLUTE MIRACLE AND YOUR BODY IS A MIND-BLOWING CREATION.

The more you live in touch with this, the kinder you will be to yourself through all of the choices you make—the food, drinks, your approach to 'beauty', the relationships you establish, and your self-talk, just to name a few.

You can accept yourself and still act to resolve health challenges. Accepting yourself doesn't mean you let the health challenges roll on. Accepting your body as it comes is one of the greatest gifts you give yourself, yet that doesn't mean you can't still practise self-care and live in the healthiest, most radiant body you can possibly live in.

There is a downside of overzealous 'self-care'. Too many teenagers and adult women are now taking self-care to detrimental levels, such as occurs in orthorexia (obsessively avoiding specific foods that they believe to be harmful) and, at times, body sculpting. You start off focused on having better health and you end up living in fear of food or overtraining. As I've mentioned, you can make consistent great-quality food choices and work out regularly from a place of genuine care for yourself, your life and your health. Or you can do those things from fear. Choose care ▪

Dr Libby Weaver

FOR THE BEAUTIFUL RADIANCE THAT COMES
FROM BEING GRATEFUL FOR THE SMALLEST
OF THINGS, WORK ON YOUR BELIEFS TO
ESTABLISH UNEQUIVOCALLY THAT YOU ARE
SO WORTH TAKING CARE OF.

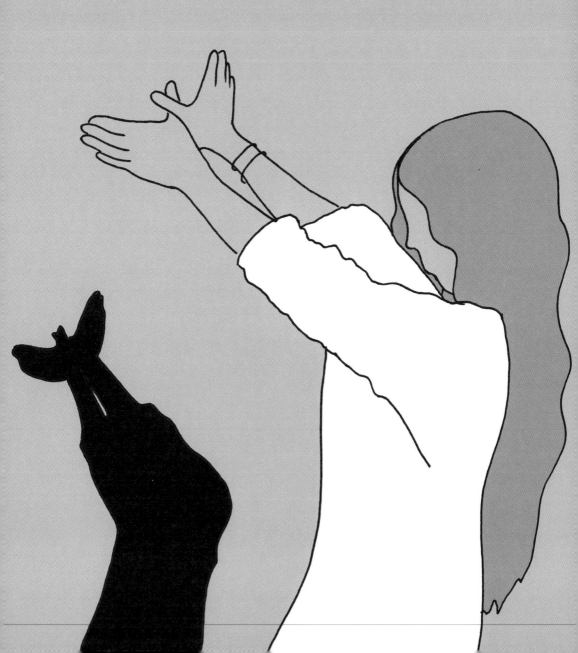

Your beauty routine

What's driving it?

I'm yet to meet someone who doesn't do this in some way. There's no right or wrong here. Just awareness to be had for us all.

When it comes to your beauty routine, ponder why you do what you do.

If you do any of the following, answer honestly why you do it. Sometimes it feels easier to be honest with others than it is with ourselves. Are these things part of your self-care routine, hiding yourself, or self-loathing? Whose approval or acceptance are you seeking? Who do you want to notice you, like you, include you or love you? If you truly need to look different to the way you do naturally for them to like you, is this person or group of people truly supposed to be in your life?

YOU DON'T HAVE TO DO ANYTHING TO BE LOVED. YOU JUST NEED TO BE YOU. YOUR BEAUTIFUL SELF. AND THE PEOPLE WHO ARE SUPPOSED TO BE IN YOUR LIFE WILL BE.

Finish this sentence. To be beautiful I need to…

Your answers might range anywhere from 'be my authentic self' or 'act with integrity' to 'have perfect hair, nails and skin' or 'never be seen without makeup'. Or maybe your list is really long. Maybe you have to look or be a certain way to appear to yourself (or others) as beautiful and, to create that, there's a lot on your list. For a participant in one of my recent women's health weekends, her list said:

To be beautiful I must:

- always be seen with makeup
- always have a tan
- ensure I keep my eyebrow shape up to date with trends
- keep up with my facial peels
- keep on top of my Botox, lip and cheek fillers
- keep in shape
- be kind
- be patient
- think of others before myself
- love everyone.

With so many things on her list—that, to your mind, all have to be happening

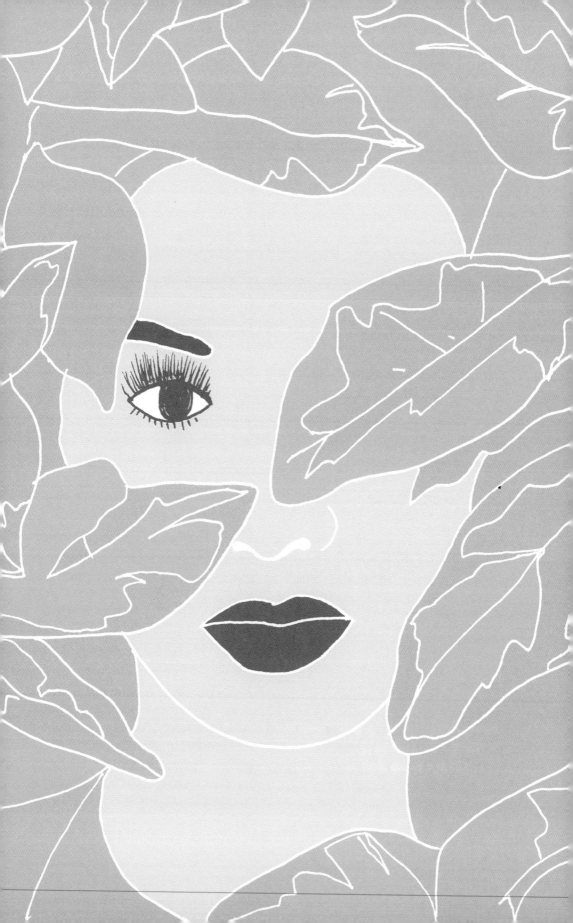

at the same time—do you think this dear lady ever felt beautiful? No. Yet for another in the room, her list said:

To be beautiful I must:

- wake up.

Now she may have meant wake up each day or wake up in the sense of the Pema Chodron quote (page 157). With only one thing on her list, which is basically about her simply existing, do you think she is radiant most days? Yes.

JUST START TO THINK ABOUT HOW YOU PERCEIVE YOUR OWN BEAUTY.

Why do you:

- wear makeup
- get spray tans
- get Botox
- have your cheeks injected
- have your lips injected
- contemplate getting breast implants
- think about getting a tummy tuck after giving birth
- get liposuction?

What are you wanting these processes or their after-effects to lead you to FEEL? Not *have*, feel? Name the feelings.

What other ways could you experience these feelings? Please don't get me wrong. I am not saying that doing any of these things is wrong. I am simply wanting you to make choices from a

place of loving yourself rather than from the false perception of your not enoughness.

Contemplate who you do these things for Is it for:

- yourself
- your boyfriend, partner or husband
- your friends
- other women
- society as a collective?

THE MASKS YOU WEAR

We all wear masks at times. And in this case, I'm not referring to any potential visible masks. I'm talking about the way we change our behaviour in different settings or company. Sometimes this is essential to keep us safe, or to keep our heart open yet protected, while other times, we mask up to ensure we are liked or accepted or to hide our true feelings or our authentic selves. It can be the ego at work, telling you that you have to be a certain way around this particular person

For example, you might have a friend who, when she isn't in a great place herself, really goes to town talking about other people and what she finds annoying about them or what's wrong with her life. Perhaps you don't enjoy this and after your interactions with her, you feel tired and awful, having joined in with her judgemental commentary. You know this isn't who you are and that you don't even agree with her stance on these oth eople or her pity party for herself. Yet hile you are in her company you wear a ask. Why? Is it so she feels better about erself? Or so she keeps you as a friend?

/hat do you think might happen if ou spoke up and let her know that ou're uncomfortable with this train of onversation and that you'd much rather lk about something that adds light to he world, not takes away from that?

)r if you gently enquired why sometimes hen you catch up she seems like he's hurting because she appears to e judging all these people and if she hurting, is she okay and can you elp in any way? It might feel scary or uncomfortable, but it breaks the walls down. That helps you both return to being your authentic selves. And that's one of the things I mean about there being so much beauty in you being your authentic self. For when you aren't, not only does growth for both of you cease but you allow fear, rather than love, to run your life.

So when it comes to your beauty, focus on singing from your heart, not a mentality that you are lacking. In anything. Radiate beauty from the depths of your soul ■

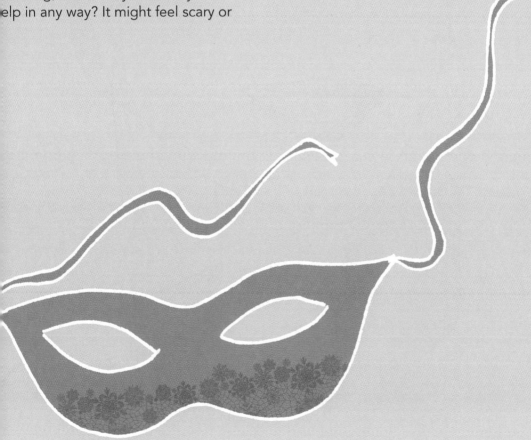

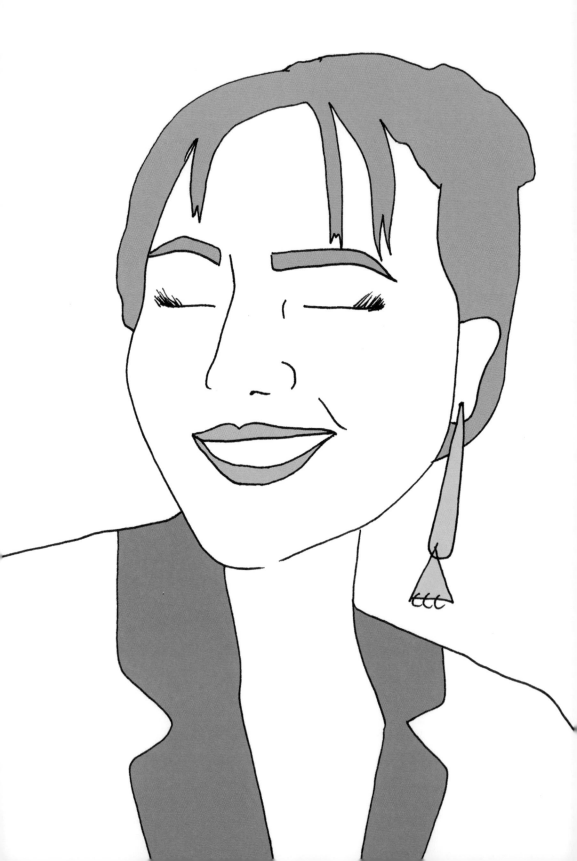

"

ACCEPT THAT ONLY YOU
ARE RESPONSIBLE FOR
YOU. YOUR FOOD, YOUR
THOUGHTS AND YOUR
ACTIONS. NO ONE ELSE
CAN DO IT FOR YOU. LET
THAT AWAKEN ENDLESS,
BEAUTIFUL POSSIBILITIES
WITHIN YOU.

"

– Dr Libby

Dr Libby Weaver

The pursuit of perfection

What's it really about?

Have you ever felt the desire or need to be perfect, either in some area of your life or across all of it? Maybe you want your appearance to look perfect, or feel a drive to portray a perfect life to others. Or, if you don't relate to this, perhaps someone immediately springs to mind who you think does all she can to appear perfect.

Whether you pursue perfection or know someone who does, let's leave all judgements at the door and peel back the layers on this to uncover what it might really be about.

Because, for some, it is a destructive path that takes away too much joy in life. And even if we aren't driven by perfection, most of us are reticent to be open about parts of our lives we feel shameful of and will instead do what we can to cover up things that we perceive might not be going so well.

STORY OF PERFECTION

Imagine a little girl. As she grows up and becomes aware of her body, she starts to perceive others are judging her appearance (refer to page 11). Life up until now has really been about her need to behave well, and this has now transferred to another department of her life—she now needs to look perfect too. When she is eight years old, this might mean having her hair in a certain style— ponytail or braids for example—or it may impact where she wants the hemline of her school uniform to fall. By the time she is 13, her pursuit of perfection might see her wanting to wear foundation to school to appear flawless, or mascara to emphasise her eyes. Also, she's been reading up on diets and started exercising because she might believe that this is the only way to keep an 'acceptably' slim figure (or perhaps estrogen has started changing the shape of her body and she fears it). Then, of course, she wants to do well at school and get good grades. Sometimes only 100 per cent on a test will do; anything else is failing, even if she tops the class.

The intensity of pressure she places on herself to be perfect, let alone the fear she lives with every day, not to mention the food restrictions that may have started by now, can lead her periods to go awry. Either heavy and painful or she stops getting them at all. And well-intentioned, concerned adults may put her on the pill. Not for contraception, but to 'regulate' her periods.

The pill stops her pituitary communicating with her ovaries and they stop making hormones, which is how the pill prevents ovulation and hence pregnancy. So, her body now relies on synthetic hormones, not identical but similar enough for her body to accept that it doesn't have to make its own any more and enough so she gets her period back.

Now with very low innate progesterone production, she's lost one of the most powerful anti-anxiety and antidepressant agents in her body. So, she feels even more stressed out. Add to that the depressant action on the nervous system that happens in anyone who has an excess of estrogen and she faces a scenario that is true for too many young girls these days—she is (well-meaningly) placed on antidepressants. So, by the time she is 16 she is on two of the world's most powerful medications—and she believes she has a disease. Even without this pill scenario, moods can fluctuate, just from the tension a teenage girl feels to be perfect.

Fast forward to her early adult years and she has either had or still has disordered eating; had or has an irritated bowel and gets bloated most days which translates in her head to 'I am fat'. She is quite obsessed with her body which gets masked by the concept that exercise and 'clean eating' are how we're supposed to look after ourselves. Her periods are all over the place, if she gets them, or she may have been diagnosed with a reproductive system condition. She questions herself at every turn and constantly worries what other people think of her. She thinks if she could just find or reach xyz, she would be so much happier. But the truth is, in focusing on her perceived flaws, in trying to achieve a perfect life, she's simply missing all of the beauty and magic and wonder that is already there around and within her.

DURING CHILDHOOD, MOST YOUNG GIRLS ARE RAISED TO BE 'GOOD GIRLS'. TO DO AS WE ARE TOLD, TO PUT THE NEEDS OF OTHERS AHEAD OF OUR OWN.

This tends to please the person (usually a parent) requesting (or demanding) this of us and their intention for us is (usually) simply to create a well-adjusted, mindful child who will grow into a thoughtful adult member of society. In some women however, this sets up pathways in the nervous system and psychology that, to be loved, we have to do everything right and can never get into trouble. So, you do all you can to be good.

nderneath this drive for perfection, what we're really looking for is to return to the day—a day you can no longer remember—when in your very essence you had certainty that you were loved unconditionally.

here is a massive difference between having an appreciation of excellence and the need to appear perfect, between having standards of self-care and not caring at all. The problem comes when you believe that to be loved, liked, appreciated, to fit in, be the best, special or the favourite, you must be, do, act and appear perfect. Which, in your own eyes, will be a never-ending, unrelenting, exhausting and futile pursuit. For you only pursue because in your heart you don't feel good enough the way that you are. here is nothing in this world that you an do, say, have or be that will make ou more perfect than you ready are ■

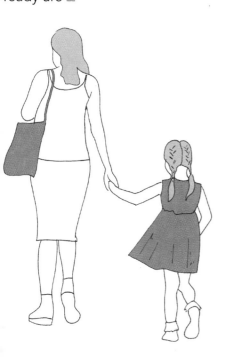

REFLECTION

At its core, the pursuit of perfection comes from wanting to be loved. If you reflect on your life, whose love did you crave the most growing up? It's almost always your mother or your father's.

Who did you perceive you had to be for this person?

Who could you never be? (1)

Imagine for a moment that your heart interviewed their heart. Do you think they want you to be perfect or happy?

Would their heart want you to be who you perceive you need to be or who you really are?

Even though the person's behaviour may have been, at times, challenging, unacceptable or even illegal, can you consider that their behaviour was the product of their joys and their pains in life? Recognising this, could you consider forgiving them—not the behaviour, but the soul behind the behaviour, with their joys and pains that shaped their interactions with you?

There is no need to pursue perfection. Drop this fearful mask. You are the perfect you, created complete just as you are. Always learning, always evolving. Live in touch with the truth and beauty of your uniqueness and shine and share the gift of you with the world.

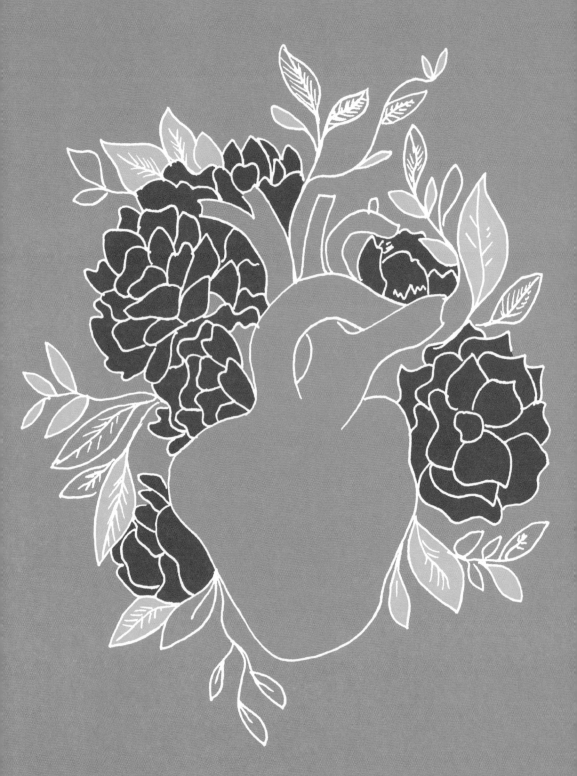

Dr Libby Weaver

Illumination

The true beauty in your heart

Never stop believing in your own radiance, even if you feel others have urged you to dim your own light. You don't stop believing in the sun when the moon comes out. You don't stop believing in the moon when the clouds pass over her face.

You may have a moment when you judge yourself harshly. You may have days or—hopefully not—weeks when you feel anything but beautiful. But never stop believing in your beauty, even if it momentarily disappears from your own view, because of choices you have made.

You are not your behaviour. You need to take responsibility for your behaviour, but you are not it. We usually behave poorly when we perceive (notice that I write 'perceive') that we have lost, or may lose, love or acceptance, or if we perceive we have let someone down or failed. But there is no failure. There's only feedback.

Be just like the sun that shines its light upon the world. Remember that you, too, light up the world with your very presence.

Beauty is a light in your heart, and it doesn't just light up your own gorgeous face; it helps light up the whole world. For when we let our own light shine, we give others permission to do the same (1). Open your eyes wide—I mean that literally—and see the wonder in the world.

Open your eyes wide, knowing that there is such beauty in your heart, and marvel at the gift that you are ∎

NEVER STOP BELIEVING IN YOURSELF OR IN LIFE.

BEAU

TY

solutions

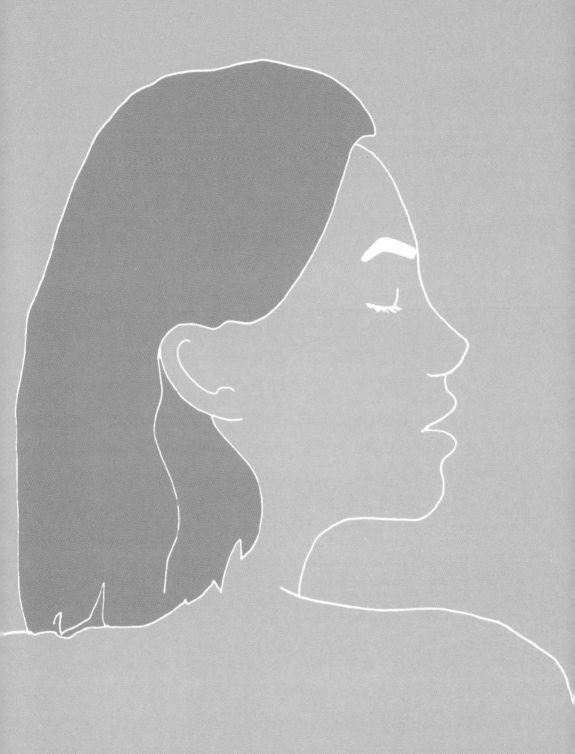

Dr Libby Weaver

Insights into beauty challenges

What is your body trying to tell you?

I am driven to help people literally get to the heart of their health matters. As you now understand, I believe that the so-called markers of beauty—such as your skin, hair and nails—are simply a barometer for inner processes. And the outer reflection of these is simply your body doing its best to wake you up to eat, drink, move, think, breathe, believe, or perceive in a different way than you're now. When you can consider an outer beauty challenge to be a gift from your body, even though that is the last thing it feels like when you are in the midst of an acute or chronic beauty challenge, it can open you up to explore this in an entirely new way.

FOR MANY PEOPLE TODAY, THERE IS A FEAR AND ANXIETY WITHIN THEM; OFTEN CENTRED ON WHETHER THEY ARE GOOD ENOUGH.

Anxious feelings can only be present if you are focused on the future.

Despondent emotions can usually only be present if you focus on the past. If you are present, there is only peace. That may sound like a cliché, however, pause to really consider this.

Dr John Demartini (1) and Louise Hay (2) teach that thoughts and beliefs you may or may not be aware of can lead to dysfunction in your physical health. This makes sense when you think that your perceptions, if loving, lead you to make more love hormones (oxytocin and serotonin for example), while if fearful, you will produce more stress hormones (adrenaline or cortisol)—even though nothing may have physically taken place. You make these hormones based on your thoughts.

Let's look at an example. Say you're thinking about your relationship with your significant other. As you drive to work you're thinking about how lovely it was that they made you breakfast this morning and how lucky you are to have such a kind and considerate partner who goes out of their way to support you. Contrast that with a time when you're thinking about how little your significant other does to help you around the house and, boy, how frustrating is it that if you don't pick up the vacuum, the house would be a swamp of dust and dirt and why can't they just think about doing this without you having to ask? Or, if you are single at the moment contrast a time when that feels like the most spacious thing in the world to a time when it feels like the most lonely thing in the world. In both of these examples, nothing has actually taken place, but they both lead you to produce very different hormones. And all of this just from your mind.

Sometimes, during a session, I would ask a client whether they felt a particular emotional state or phrase resonated for them, based on the work of aforementioned authors, or my own intuition. I often found that the client did feel a certain way or that the phrase did speak to her, and this led us to an insight that often had a wonderful impact across many areas of her life. Once you catch a glimpse of a belief that you created to help you make sense of a situation, often a long time ago, you see that it is just something you made up! You can't un-see that. So, life changes in a great way and a part of you feels freer.

WITH LESS STRESS HORMONE OUTPUT, THE BODY CAN HEAL AND REGULATE ITSELF FAR MORE EASILY.

An example of how food and beliefs interact is graciously demonstrated in the case of an eight-year-old girl (who I will call Beth) who I worked with a few years ago. Beth's mother brought her to see me as most of the child's body was covered in eczema. For her age, Beth was quite small in size. However, she ate 12 pieces of fruit each day! Just as an aside, that's far too much for an adult, let alone a child!

Many fruits are naturally high in phenolic compounds which help to give them flavour. The liver has to make an enzyme called phenol-sulphur transferase to detoxify (change) aspects of these substances and sometimes the liver can't keep up with demands. Two pieces a day is no problem for most people, but 12! That's a lot to ask of a small bodied eight year-old.

To that end, I asked Beth and her mother to reduce the fruit consumption to five pieces per day—still too many but I didn't want to reduce it further as I didn't want her losing weight, given that she was already quite tiny. When they came back four weeks later, the eczema had improved, but it was not resolving in the way it does when the dietary change has nailed it, when it has gotten to the heart of the reaction. I felt there was something else at play. Sure, we could reduce the fruit more (while we ensured Beth ate other foods instead), but I wasn't convinced this scenario was all dietary. In children with eczema, I have seen (the right) dietary change for

hat child completely resolve eczema in
ight weeks. The redness goes out of
 in 10 days when you are on the right
ack and then it can take a few weeks
or the skin to heal. As an aside, the
elta-6-desaturase (an enzyme) content
f evening primrose oil, as well as its
amma-linolenic acid (GLA) content,
ssists with the skin healing, allowing
t to be incorporated into the skin,
ourishing it and making it soft and
upple again.

eth's mum actually raised the emotional
spect with me, saying she'd explained
 Beth that she might like to do some
olouring-in, in the (safe) reception area,
hile Beth's mum and I talked. Beth's
um knew of the third pillar of my work
nd asked me if I thought it was playing a
le in Beth's skin. I shared that, according
 the work of Dr Demartini (1) and
ouise Hay (2), eczema was 'rage at a
asculine presence' and in someone as
oung as Beth, it was likely to be Dad; so
enquired about Beth's relationship with
er father. Beth's mum shared with me
at he was a loving father, but that she
ouldn't be surprised if Beth didn't feel
eeply loved by him. I enquired as to why
nd she went on to explain.

eth is the middle child with an older
ister and a younger brother. Her older
ister is tall and physically strong and into
port, while her younger brother is playful
nd also loves sport. Beth is physically
mall and her passions are art and drama.

When Dad wanted to go for a bike ride,
he often only asked the older sister, not
Beth, as he'd said Beth couldn't keep
up. When Dad wanted to kick a football,
he'd take the younger brother to the
park and not invite Beth. Beth's mum was
also planning a trip to visit family in the
UK and in a conversation between the
parents in the kitchen one night, Beth's
dad had asked Beth's mum to take Beth
with her as he 'couldn't handle' her. Beth
had overheard this conversation. So,
although Beth's father was asking her
mother to take Beth to the UK out of love
for Beth (as she was closer to her mother
and they had more in common and she
would therefore be happier there with
her mum than at home with him), to
Beth all of this would have potentiated
the subconscious story that her dad didn't
love her.

As the realisation of this hit Beth's mum
she was mortified for Beth and her
husband and knew he would be too.
But she wanted to see if a change in their
relationship could help her daughter's
skin. She knew Beth's dad would be
open to that too, as he loved all his
children very much. I suggested that the
dad come up with what to do as I felt it
needed to be an authentic expression of
his love to truly connect with Beth and
heal her heart. With this in mind, they
went home with the intention to see me
again four weeks later.

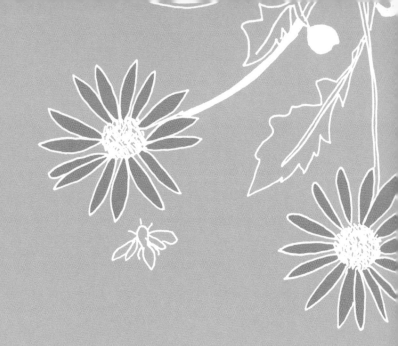

LIFE HAPPENS
FOR YOU,
NOT TO YOU.

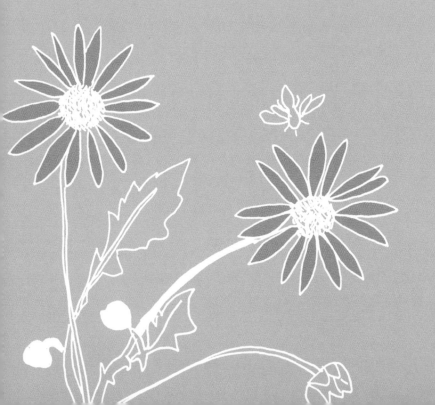

ere's what happened in those four eeks.

eth's mum explained to her husband hat Beth likely perceived to be her ther's lack of love. He very much anted to correct this perception and emonstrate his love for her in a way at was meaningful to her. Beth was the ad in the school play and the family had ttended on opening night. On the final ight of the play, Beth's mum went to pick er up. Being from the UK, and from a mily who had a theatrical background, ey were all aware (Beth included) of e tradition to make a fuss of the lead n closing night. Something they used o do within the family but had let go f in recent years. Beth and her mother rrived home after closing night to a dark ouse. However, as soon as they came rough the front door, the lights flashed n and there in front of Beth was her ther, sister and brother, with bunting nd signs saying 'Congratulations Beth'. his arms, her father held an enormous unch of flowers, almost as tall as Beth. e crouched down, handed them to her, ssed her cheek and smiled broadly as e said congratulations and kind words o her. She simply said thank you, and en said she needed to have her shower. nd off she scurried. A while later she merged wearing her pyjamas and alked into the lounge room where her other and father were sitting. Without word she climbed up on her father's p, curled herself up into a tiny ball and bbed and sobbed and sobbed.

Four weeks later, back they came for me to see Beth—and there was virtually no trace of eczema. I could make out a small patch of dry skin (not red or raised) on her arm but the rest of her skin was clear and smooth. Everyone was thrilled. I get covered in goosebumps and my eyes brim with tears every time I reflect on Beth's experience.

I can't tell you if it was just more time on five (instead of 12) pieces of fruit a day that resolved Beth's eczema, or if it was correcting her perception that her father didn't love her, or if it was the synergy of both of these changes.

FOR ME, THIS IS PRECIOUS EVIDENCE OF THE WAY OUR FOOD AND PERCEPTIONS CO-CREATE OUR HEALTH AND THAT THE BODY IS A MAGNIFICENT VEHICLE OF COMMUNICATION IF WE CAN LEARN TO DECIPHER HER MESSAGES.

Thank goodness for the open-heartedness of Beth's mum and dad, for their daughter now gets to grow up with a different diet, which even after all of my years of working in nutrition, pales in significance to what a change in perception, to what a return to the truth, offers us and our health. It's breathtaking.

Life happens for you, not to you. I know we can't always get resolution on things that have happened in our lives in the past (the way Beth did with her dad), but there is always an opportunity to explore our beliefs and to consider that they were created in response to our perception of events rather than how things actually were. That way, we can explore what happened with fresh, adult eyes, instead of living with the meaning we created as a child about what the 'what happened' meant.

For example, if a teenage girl with an eating disorder says to me, 'Dad left because he didn't love me', part of her healing begins when she discovers that a lack of love for her was not even an inkling of a contributing factor to him leaving.

In this section, I share some skin and other conditions with you to show you how they might be explored from a dietary and emotional perspective.

Please understand that there are almost always physical processes such as dietary change that need to occur for these skin conditions to heal. And for many people, dietary change is all they need.

However, for some people dietary change generates significant improvements but not a complete resolution. So I am offering the emotional information for those who may need the emotional insight in order for their skin (or other) challenge to resolve. If any of the concepts resonate for you, consider it an opportunity to enquire within.

Perhaps use a journal, and explore whether these perceptions still serve you or whether they are based on a story you made up a long time ago about who you are or who you had to be to be loved, or who you could never be. If the emotional approach is not for you, or doesn't ring true for you, simply consider the dietary and nutritional ideas.

Explore both if you can for the best results.

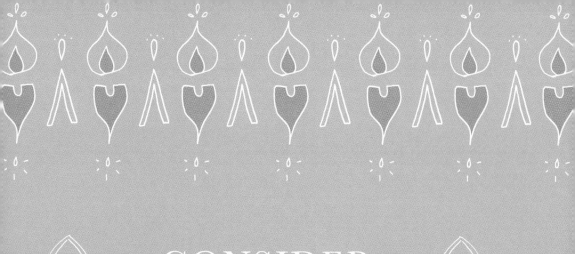

CONSIDER
HOW YOU
EAT
DRINK
MOVE
THINK
BREATHE
BELIEVE
OR
PERCEIVE

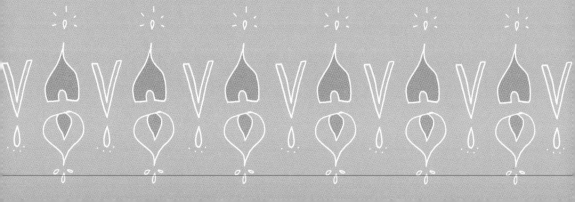

Nutritional

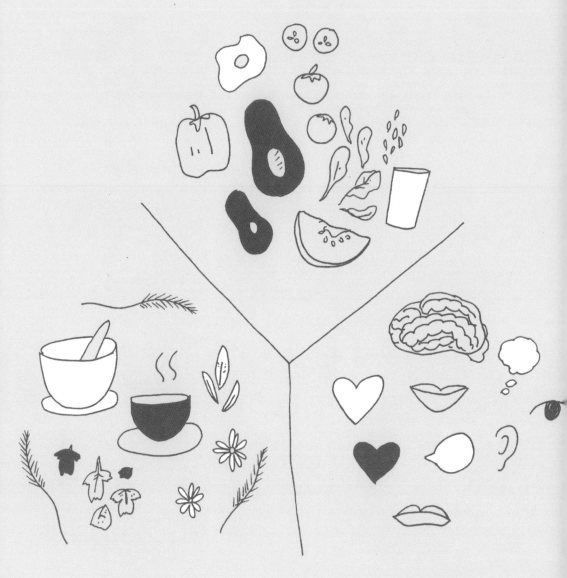

Herbal

Emotional

Beauty solutions

Solving your frustrations from the inside out

You now understand that beauty really is an inside job. Without great quality food full of nutrients and antioxidants as well as hydration, our digestion, liver and kidney function, plus our sex hormone balance, are all going to become compromised. As a result, the skin and other beauty bits can suffer, creating frustration and sadness for you in the process.

Remember, too, that the beauty bits can be compromised when stress hormones are being churned out. When this happens, non-vital processes such as the clarity of your skin, nail strength, and hair, brow and eyelash lush factor, are not deemed important to your survival when you are on red alert.

This is my take on what I have seen work for some common 'beauty' challenges—nutritional, herbal and emotional. Here, I simply offer a guide and recommend that you explore within yourself what feels true or right for you. Not every pathway will work for every single person, although a change in diet to include an abundance of vegetables is a fantastic starting point for everyone.

My knowledge of biochemistry and my clinical experience has taught me that in

order to find the road to healing, we have to find the route we took to create the problem.

This just means if it is a zinc deficiency at the heart of your skin and weak nail issue, correcting this deficiency by increasing your zinc levels through diet or supplementation will be the solution. But also remember that the body isn't always so simple.

WE HAVE TO FIND THE ROUTE WE TOOK TO CREATE THE PROBLEM.

Perhaps it is a deficiency of zinc, but maybe also your digestion isn't optimal and so you're not absorbing the zinc that you start to consume to correct the problem. So digestive system support work in this scenario would also be needed. Or there might be an emotional aspect for you to explore, and until you do, no amount of dietary change will correct the problem because what your body is guiding you to explore and understand is a past hurt or a belief that you're holding on to. I've also found that the solution we are most resistant to exploring is often the one that will lead to the greatest change. For example, if the idea of taking a break from coffee or alcohol or gluten or sugar for a few short weeks of your very long life feels particularly difficult, chances are you will find it is a big part of the solution. We are all a bit funny like that.

All of this is simply to say don't give up hope if you don't find the solution immediately. And have the courage to explore what feels like even the most challenging solutions to you.

REMEMBER ALSO THAT THINGS TAKE TIME.

You can't always expect to see change in a week, particularly if it's been something that's been challenging for you for years. Sometimes we need to focus on re-establishing solid foundations before we will see the changes we seek take effect. I can't emphasise this enough.

Having read the section about the skin, how it functions and the importance of allowing it to be the radiant organ it was designed to be, you may also feel inspired to support your skin and overall health more by changing what you put on your skin.

Instead of spending a fortune working

from the outside in, focus some of those resources on moving towards an inside-out focus.

This might involve nourishing yourself with more organic produce and fewer skin 'care' products that either add a load to your detoxification mechanisms, disturb the function of the skin (such as disrupting the acid mantle and its ability to offer protection from bacterial penetration, which helps prevent pimples and acne) and/or have troublesome consequences on other species or the aquatic environment. When you think about your body, or a specific part that you struggle to accept, ask yourself how you can best 'nourish' this part of you, and see what your heart offers you as a suggestion.

Some of the solutions offered here you will have seen throughout the book already, but I list them here, in one place to give you a quick reference guide.

At the end, I've put together a list of common beauty challenges and some of the specific solutions I've found to be effective over the years.

Please note that any dietary changes are best guided by an experienced nutrition professional who can ensure you aren't missing any key nutrients. Taking herbal medicine is best directed by a medical herbalist. If you struggle to gain insight into your emotions on your own, or if doing so may cause significant distress, seeing a counsellor or psychologist can be highly beneficial.

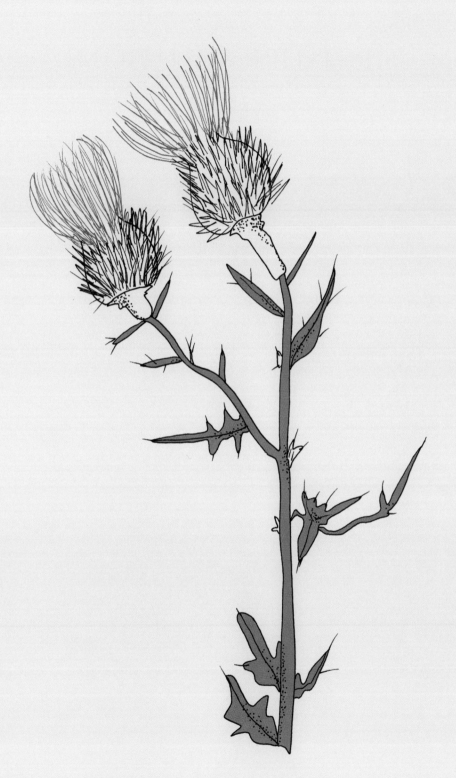

St Mary's thistle

FIRST-TIER SOLUTIONS

These are the simplest solutions that virtually everyone would benefit from applying because they lay the foundation for great health. And, as you now understand, we need excellent health to look and feel our best.

INCREASE PLANT INTAKE

I've said this already a number of times, but I can't emphasise the importance of it enough. It truly is nutrients that keep us alive. The minerals they contain support longevity and the antioxidants slow premature ageing. When you eat plenty of plants, the waste-removal systems of the body also obtain what they need for efficient functioning, which also bodes well for your skin and overall health. Don't just think of vegetables as a token effort on the side of your plate at dinner. Make them the centre of your meal and add other things to them. If you struggle with inspiration or ideas, there is an abundance of high-plant recipes online or on my website: drlibby.com.

INCREASE GENTLE MOVEMENT

Such as walking, rebounding, tai chi, qi gong and yoga to support natural lymphatic flow. This is particularly important for addressing cellulite and skin challenges as good lymphatic flow supports efficient movement of waste away from cells to be disposed of.

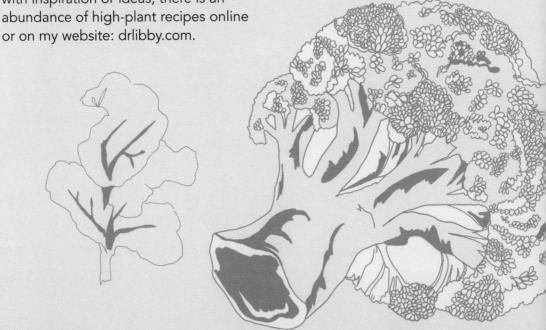

ADDRESS YOUR BREATHING

Diaphragmatic breathing is how we communicate safety to our body; it is how our body recognises that we aren't in danger and ensures that all our body systems are functioning optimally. Truly, the ripple effect of consistent long, slow breaths is major and so positive for so many aspects of your wellbeing. Put your hands on the bottom of your ribcage just below your sternum and feel if you're breathing diaphragmatically right now. It will feel like this area expands with your inhalation and deflates with your exhalation. If you don't feel this section moving, bring your awareness to where your breath is moving—it will most likely be your upper chest. It is usually adrenaline driving this way of breathing, which (when we don't need to be escaping from danger) brings with it its host of problematic consequences that you've learnt about throughout the book, including whether we can efficiently use body fat as a fuel or not. The more you diaphragmatically breathe, the more relaxed and calm your body (and body systems) will be. So, if it's something you need to work on, make a daily commitment to a breathing practice or a breath-focused movement practice such as Stillness Through Movement, tai chi, yoga or Pilates. The more you breathe in a way that communicates safety to your body, the more your body will naturally transition to breathing this way over time.

REDUCE LIVER LOADERS

Eat whole, real foods only. Cut out refined sugar and anything artificial including sweeteners, flavours, colours, preservatives. Significantly reduce or eliminate caffeine and alcohol from your lifestyle for at least three months. This also includes only putting products on your skin that aren't synthetic and are ideally organic. If cutting some of these things out of your lifestyle feels challenging for you, turn it into a challenge! See how long you can go without them. Or start by significantly reducing them and work towards cutting them out. And remember, it doesn't have to be forever—just take a break to reduce the load on your detoxification pathways for a while. Do what feels comfortable for you and then stretch a little further.

MAKE WATER YOUR MAIN DRINK

No soft drink, reconstituted juice or cordial at all. If you feel like something fizzy or sweet, pour a glass of sparkling water with some freshly cut fruit. Kombucha is another delicious and refreshing alternative and as a fermented product, it is beneficial for your gut health. Just make sure you choose a low-sugar option. Look at the label and make sure it has less than 5 grams of sugar per 100mL.

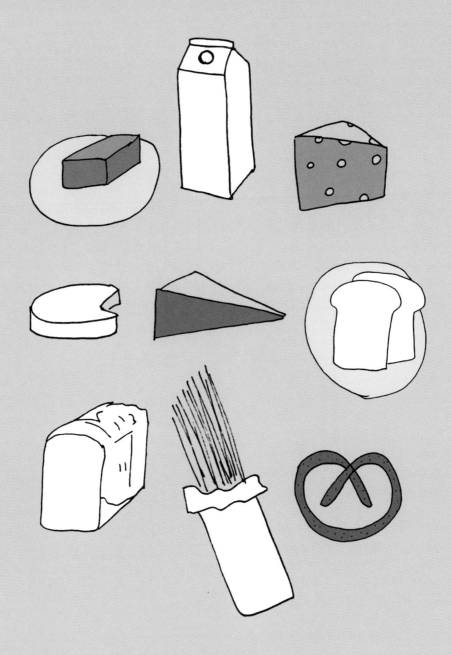

Dr Libby Weaver

SECOND-TIER SOLUTIONS

If the first-tier solutions haven't been enough to initiate change, this is the next step to take. Again, it's not to suggest that you take them all (or all at once), only that I have seen them effectively help to heal beauty challenges that people have come to see me about over the years.

TRIAL A DAIRY-FREE DIET FOR A MINIMUM OF TWO MONTHS

This means all dairy foods as well as foods that contain dairy products that you may not suspect they are in, such as salt and vinegar chips (although if you have already applied tier one strategies, these won't be part of your daily life!). See an experienced nutrition professional to ensure all nutrient requirements are being met if you find that it makes a difference and decide to continue to eat this way beyond the two-month trial. From a dietary perspective in this second-tier of change, this is the approach I've seen have the most noticeable positive effect on skin in particular. In my experience, an indication that you may respond well to this change is if you have a history of streptococcus-based infections such as tonsillitis (strep throat), ear infections, chest infection, bronchitis, sinus infections, or if you have trouble breathing through your nose and instead you mostly breathe through your mouth. Or if you have or have had eczema and/or asthma.

TRIAL A GLUTEN-FREE DIET FOR TWO MONTHS

In my experience, this is warranted if you have Irish heritage, have a history of or currently have gut problems such as intermittent bouts of diarrhoea and constipation, and/or an autoimmune disease. Notice if your skin improves when eating this way. Just as with dairy-free, if you trial this, it needs to be strict for the trial period. If it doesn't make a difference to your skin after a strict two-month trial without it, you can bring gluten-containing foods back. If you continue to eat this way beyond the two-month trial, it would be wise to consult a nutrition professional to ensure all of your nutritional needs are being met.

REDUCE FRUIT CONSUMPTION

If you currently eat more than four pieces a day and particularly if you are wanting to address bumps under your skin or on the top of your arms, you may notice improvements if you reduce your fruit consumption to a maximum of two pieces per day. Or if you also have gut problems such as bloating, try eating fruit only on an empty stomach first thing in the morning to see if that makes a difference. Don't get me wrong. Fruit is highly nutritious and is rich in a number of antioxidants. Some people simply overconsume it or their gut ferments some of the substances in fruit in a way that disrupts other processes working optimally.

TRIAL A LOW FODMAP WAY OF EATING

If you noticed your skin went haywire around the same time you started to suffer with irritable bowel syndrome (IBS) type symptoms, you may like to trial a low FODMAP way of eating. This way of eating reduces specific substances in food that ferment in a way that causes problems for some people. It must be guided by a nutrition professional experienced in a low FODMAP way of eating as, for a period of time, it excludes many fruits and vegetables and you need to ensure your nutritional needs are being met.

STRESS MANAGEMENT

As discussed throughout the book, stress hinders the optimal functioning of many body systems as well as the visible 'beauty bits'. The way to reduce stress hormone production is different for everyone as a wide variety of things can trigger stress hormone production. For you it might be your email inbox or trying to get your children ready for school, whereas for someone else it might be comments on social media or what other people think of them. Generally, strategies that benefit most people include reducing caffeine intake (as caffeine leads the body to produce adrenaline), exploring our perception of pressure and urgency, as well as activating the calm arm of the nervous system via diaphragmatic breathing. Additional tips are listed on page 146. I encourage you to apply those that most resonate for you

FEEL IT IN YOUR BODY

Always notice how your body responds to your choices—to what you say, how you behave and decisions you make. Our minds can make up stories to justify all sorts of things (we all do this), yet the body does not lie. Tune into the gifts of insight she offers you.

Please note that a low FODMAP diet is not designed to be followed long term.

EXPLORE YOUR EMOTIONAL LANDSCAPE

Use the strategies offered in this book to explore your relationship with yourself, the beliefs you may have around your own self-worth and any experiences that may have instilled a sense deep inside of you that you aren't enough just as you are.

Some examples to help you begin to explore this include:

If your skin is red, inflamed, or flushes easily, or you notice these symptoms occur only at certain times, consider if you feel angry easily. And does this anger mask a sadness that you might be able to explore (with a caring friend or experienced psychologist)?

If you notice that you retain fluid or experience constipation, explore if you are finding it difficult to let go of something or someone. Often our mind comes up with all sorts of fear-based reasons to cling tightly when deep in our heart we know when a letting go is needed. Sometimes we might worry that letting go will be hurtful (to us and/or a loved one); however, we can do our best to make it gentle if that is preferred. Courage and trust are often traits that serve us well as we move through such times.

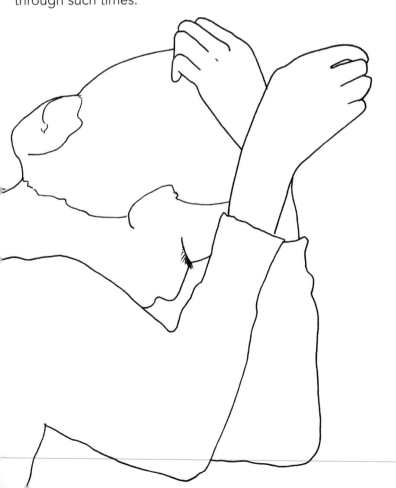

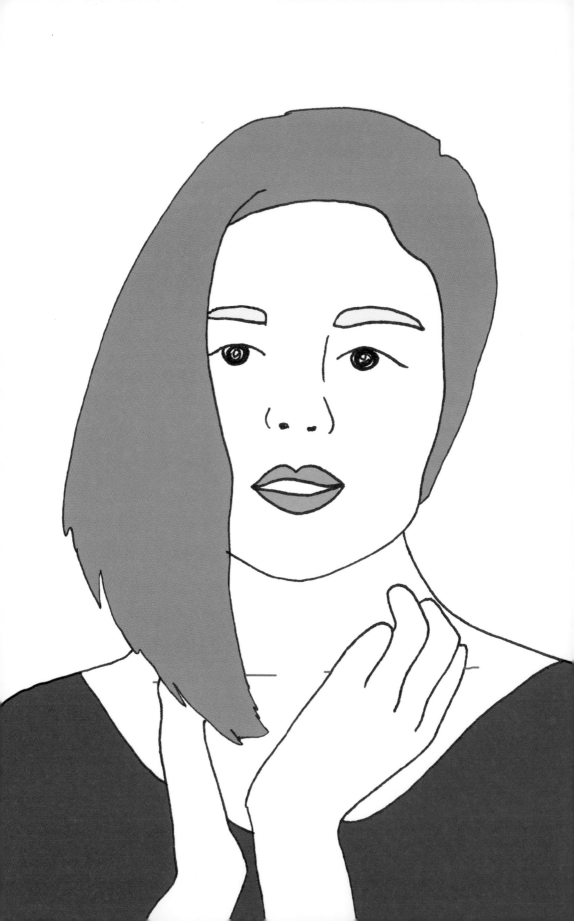

"
The only lasting beauty is

THE BEAUTY
OF THE
HEART.

"

— Rumi

SUPPLEMENTS AND HERBAL MEDICINE THAT MAY HELP

Consider taking a food-based zinc supplement to support skin healing.

Taking liver herbs to support the efficient clearance of sex hormones from the body. These might include St Mary's thistle, globe artichoke, turmeric, bupleurum, gentian and/or dandelion. A number of these also support the lymphatic system.

You may notice that changes in your skin are linked to your menstrual cycle. For example:

- If you don't get your periods regularly, herbal medicine may be beneficial. Combining the herbs paeonia and licorice (particularly for women with polycystic ovarian syndrome or PCOS), or taking chaste tree (vitex) can be helpful. It can be wise to work with a nutritionist or medical herbalist to assist you in establishing a regular cycle.

- If your periods are heavy, clotty and painful it may be due to an excess of estrogen in the second half of the menstrual cycle (in the lead-up to menstruation). You want to support your body to clear 'used up' estrogen from the body, and supporting the liver is the best way to do this. Refer to page 88 for more information

about this and/or utilise the liver herb mentioned above for a minimum of two menstrual cycles.

DHA is an omega-3 fatty acid and an essential fatty acid (EFA) that is highly beneficial to skin appearance, smoothness, radiance and overall health.

- If EFAs are supplemented, including evening primrose oil in the mix can be helpful for all skin conditions too, particularly dry skin and eczema.

Consider taking additional vitamin C as it is a wonderful antioxidant and needed for (among other processes) collagen production and to prevent collagen breakdown.

Grape seed extract is also highly beneficial for the skin. It is a potent antioxidant and, when combined with vitamin C and zinc, has been shown to reduce visible signs of ageing (3).

Including an organic green vegetable powder can be a great and simple way to boost your antioxidant intake. Add a scoop to water or your favourite green, vegetable-rich smoothie.

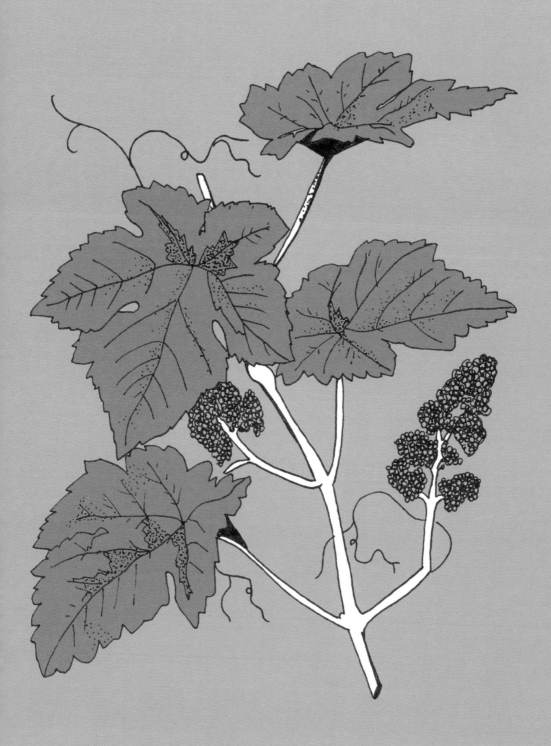

Grape seed

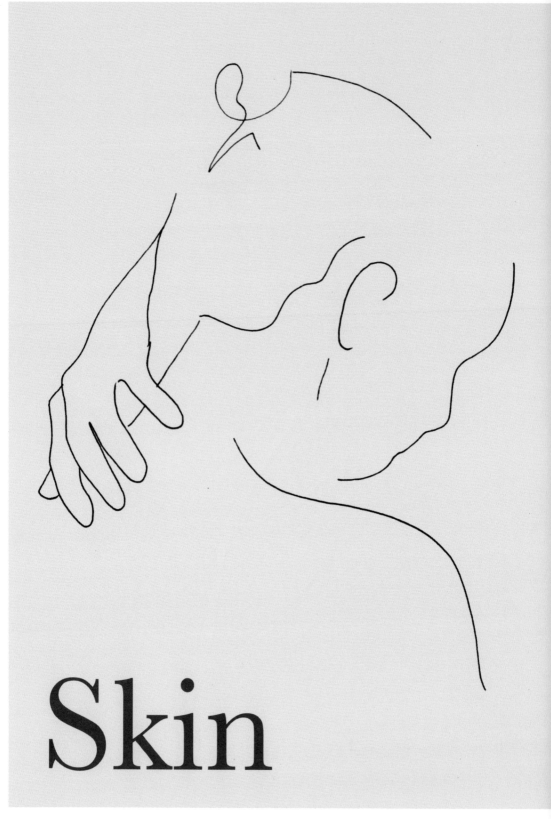

Skin

Dr Libby Weaver

Acne and back-ne

Refer to page 59 for detailed information about acne. General ideas for help with both conditions are below.

Nutrition and herbal medicine considerations

Acne is quite often perpetuated by a sex hormone imbalance arising from high levels of androgens in the skin (or in general), elevated prolactin (made by the pituitary), or an imbalance between estrogen and progesterone.

All of these situations can be tested for if the condition is ongoing or if it doesn't respond to the sex hormone balancing suggestions shared throughout the book, including liver support.

After dietary change and liver support, the next place I suggest focusing on is stress management (adrenal focus), due to the role cortisol plays in altering sex hormone conversions (see page 65 for the flow chart that shows this).

Chronic stress (among other factors) can also contribute to insulin resistance, which means that cells in the body become less responsive to the hormone insulin. Our bodies respond to this by producing more insulin, leading to elevated insulin levels.

This, in turn, stimulates androgen production which can contribute to acne.

This mechanism often affects women with PCOS.

- Eat whole, real foods only. Cut out refined sugar and anything artificial including sweeteners, flavours, colours, preservatives.

- Make water your main drink. No soft drinks at all.

- Dairy-free diet trial for a minimum of two months (with acne, three months is often needed) to break the cycle between sex hormones driving excess sebum production and the bacteria feeding on this. See an experienced nutrition professional to ensure all nutrient requirements are being met if you find that it makes a difference and continue to eat this way beyond the two to three months. Please note, you will likely notice an improvement after one month, feedback that you are on the right track.

- Consider taking a food-based zinc supplement.

- Consider taking liver herbs to support the efficient clearance of sex hormones from the body.

- Stress management is almost always needed for this too (refer to page 146).

Emotions or beliefs to explore

- Insecurity and silent anger about the perception that people are talking about you (or perhaps behind your back). Remember you can never control what other people think or say about you.

- Explore whether you have a tendency (usually inside your own mind) to make yourself feel superior—you talk yourself up—and then you quickly follow that with putting yourself down, or trash talking yourself.

Body odour

Nutrition and herbal medicine considerations

- This is usually a call for additional liver support; refer to page 91 for information about how to love your liver some more.

- Ensure you are using your bowels each day.

- Focus on eating whole, real food.

- Drink plenty of water.

Bumps on backs of arms

Nutrition and herbal medicine considerations

This can be the result of:

- An essential fatty acid (EFA) deficiency.

- Excess fruit consumption.

I've also seen it resolve with zinc supplementation. If EFAs are supplemented, including evening primrose oil in the mix can be helpful.

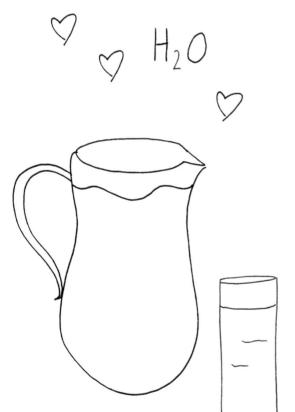

H_2O

Cellulite

Nutrition and herbal medicine considerations

- Focus on liver and lymphatic support (refer to page 91 for liver love ideas). This may include herbs such as St Mary's thistle and globe artichoke.

- Rebound to stimulate the lymphatic system—or apply any of the other strategies listed earlier.

- Significantly limiting or omitting liver loaders may also help to reduce the appearance of cellulite or, in some cases, allows it to disappear.

- Addressing estrogen dominance is also usually critical to improvements, which usually requires dietary changes specific to the individual. Common ones include an eight-week trial that involves not consuming processed foods, dairy foods and alcohol. It is also sometimes necessary to be caffeine-free during this trial.

Emotions or beliefs to explore

- Stored anger and self-punishment (2).

- You focus on where you are under-supported and forget to look for ways where you are well supported.

Cold sores

Nutrition and herbal medicine considerations

Caused by the herpes virus, so immune support is vital. Consider using:

- Additional vitamin C.

- Zinc.

- Immune support herbs can be useful, such as astragalus.

Herpes only reactivates itself when it is triggered—usually by stress, poor dietary choices, excessive sun exposure, or too little sleep. Herpes is like a seed in a desert. It will stay asleep indefinitely if the signal to germinate isn't given.

It is also important to minimise intake of foods that can feed viruses, such as reducing dietary exposure to the amino acid arginine. When the amino acid lysine is higher in your diet than the amino acid arginine, the herpes virus has trouble replicating. When arginine is higher than lysine, herpes multiplies quickly. Foods high in arginine include tree nuts as well as peanuts, seeds and chocolate. Foods high in lysine include meat, fish, eggs and legumes.

Emotions or beliefs to explore

- Festering angry words and fear of expressing them (2).

- Bitter words left unspoken (2).

"

TO BE YOURSELF
IN A WORLD THAT IS
CONSTANTLY TRYING TO
MAKE YOU SOMETHING
ELSE IS THE GREATEST
ACCOMPLISHMENT.

"

– *Ralph Waldo Emerson*

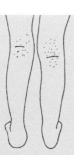

Eczema in adults

Nutrition and herbal medicine considerations

- Trial a strict dairy-free way of eating for four weeks. If that doesn't make a difference at all, bring dairy back.

- The next trial involves omitting all red foods, such as chillies, capsicums (peppers), tomatoes, strawberries, apples (red and green), for a four-week trial and see if that makes a difference.

- Or, if you eat more than two pieces of fruit a day, cut back to less than two, or omit fruit for a trial period of four weeks to see if that makes a difference.

- An evening primrose oil supplement can also be highly beneficial, as it contains gamma-linolenic acid (GLA). People with eczema are thought to be deficient in an enzyme called delta-6-desaturase, which allows fat to be incorporated into the skin, keeping it moist and youthful. The enzyme is needed to convert linoleic acid into GLA, which is why GLA appears to benefit the skin of those with eczema (atopic dermatitis).

Emotions or beliefs to explore

- Rage towards a masculine figure in your life.

- Erupting emotions (1).

- A feeling of unrelenting antagonism (1, 2).

- Chronic anxiety (try to explore what fear/s is/are behind the anxiety).

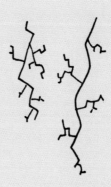

Dry skin

Nutrition and herbal medicine considerations

This may indicate:

- An EFA deficiency.

- Poor skincare choice.

- Thyroid dysfunction.

- Poor-quality diet, i.e. too much processed food and not enough real, nutrient-dense foods.

- A diet too low in fat.

- Poor digestion.

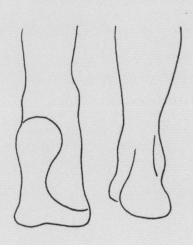

Cracked elbows or heels

Nutrition and herbal medicine considerations

This may indicate:

- An EFA deficiency.
- Zinc deficiency.

Rubbing coconut oil into elbows and heels can also assist.

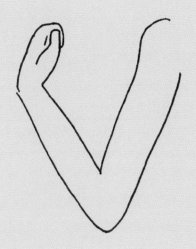

Cysts

(on or under the skin)

Nutrition and herbal medicine considerations

Be sure to have any cysts checked by your GP if they are persistent. If you get cysts on or under your skin, do a dairy-free diet trial for four weeks initially to see if that begins to make a difference. If you notice very few or no new cysts have formed, you are likely on the right track so continue the dairy-free trial for a total of three months. This means all dairy products, not just milk. If it makes no difference, the dairy can come back. If it clears it up and you want to continue with this new way of eating, consult an experienced nutrition professional to ensure you are obtaining all of the nutrients you need to stay healthy and full of energy. It is also important to take a break from processed foods and to amp up your vegetable intake, particularly greens—a minimum of five serves of vegetables every day.

If you notice that you only get cysts in the lead-up to your period, apply the sex hormone balancing strategies discussed throughout the book—considering the liver, adrenals and pituitary gland.

Emotions or beliefs to explore

Continuing to tell yourself an outdated story about something that happened in the past. Remember you now have an opportunity to see this situation with fresh, adult eyes.

Fluid accumulation at the ankles

Nutrition and herbal medicine considerations

This can indicate that the liver and/or the kidneys need support. Do a four-week trial omitting caffeine; most people will notice a significant improvement in this time. If no improvements occur, it is best to have this investigated by your GP.

Emotions or beliefs to explore

- What (or who) are you resisting letting go of?
- What (or who) are you worried about losing? (2)
- Stuck thinking; you can't see (or don't want to look for) another way.

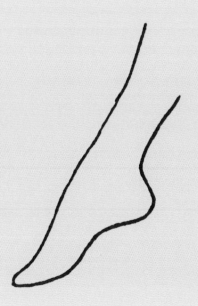

Newly oily skin or oily scalp

Nutrition and herbal medicine considerations

If greasy skin or a greasy scalp is new for you, it may signal that your sex hormones are imbalanced.

This is particularly likely to be the case if you notice the greasiness increases in the lead-up to menstruation.

Utilise the sex hormone support strategies (including liver, adrenal and pituitary support) discussed throughout the book to see if that makes a difference.

Pale, grey-tinged, dull skin

Nutrition and herbal medicine considerations

- This can be a sign of poor nutrition from poor food choices, or poor digestion.
- Focus on eating more real food, particularly plenty of vegetables, if you don't already, and/or support your digestion through stress management and the other digestion strategies suggested throughout the book.

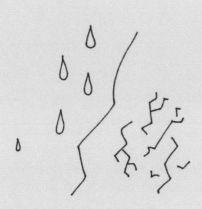

Oily and dry skin at the same time

Nutrition and herbal medicine considerations

- Work on supporting sex hormone production. In particular, make sure that the pituitary gland is talking to the ovaries and that ovulation is occurring. Paeonia and licorice or chaste tree (vitex) can offer lovely support, as can applying the strategies you discovered to help your endocrine and nervous systems feel safe (refer to page 127).

- Combination skin (dry/normal in some areas, oily in others) can also be a sign that the liver needs some love.

- Skincare may need to be changed to better support the skin's functioning. Refer to page 237 for more on ingredients to avoid.

Pimples and blemishes

Nutrition and herbal medicine considerations

Where the blemishes tend to arise can offer insight into which body system needs support. TCM practitioners are usually skilled in this. I discuss it in my book *Beauty from the Inside Out* too. For example, if blemishes always seem to appear along your jawline, it can be a sign that your sex hormones need support. Most pimples and blemishes respond well to a whole food, real food way of eating, as well as doing a dairy-free trial for four weeks. See the four weeks as an initial trial period (or it may be all you need with pimples and blemishes). If you notice your skin improving, you may like to continue for another two to three months before trialling a reintroduction. Please consult a nutrition professional to ensure all your nutrient needs are being met.

Emotions or beliefs to explore

- Intense, small outbursts of anger (2).

- What's *really* bothering you?

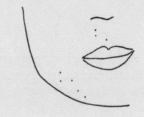

Pigmentation on face

(newly appearing)

Nutrition and herbal medicine considerations

- This can indicate a sex hormone imbalance, usually too much estrogen. Liver support can be highly worthwhile.

- It is common for pigmentation to become visible for some women while they are taking the OCP. They either usually swap from the combined pill to a progestogen only pill or they come off OCPs entirely.

- Other than the result of excessive sun exposure, new pigmentation can also be a stress response of the body with the melanocytes that sit just under the surface, switching on their production of melanin as a form of defence to a trigger or pollutants. Therefore, adrenal care, stress management and plenty of antioxidants are also important to help prevent further pigmentation appearing.

Emotions or beliefs to explore

- Did the pigmentation begin in earnest not long after a shock? Sometimes a shock can take an obvious form, while other times it might be an injury—you broke your wrist for example—and there was a shock factor in that for you, perhaps from the way you fell. Or it may be a shock that something you took for granted suddenly changed. Did you create a belief as a result of this? Perhaps 'People can't be trusted' or 'Everyone betrays me' or 'People always take advantage of me' (in relationships or in business, for example) and pause to consider if these statements are really true. For when we apply a statement that may apply to one or a small number of people to all people, your brain starts to look for evidence to back you up in your belief. Be gentle with yourself and do your best to unravel a belief that may have formed. Apply what you leant in the Am I Safe? exercises on page 127 so you can take steps in your life or belief systems to ensure you feel safe.

- Need to protect yourself from being seen, noticed or exposed too much (1).

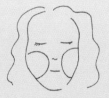

Redness on the face; flush easily

Nutrition and herbal medicine considerations

- Commit to a dairy-free diet trial for four weeks.

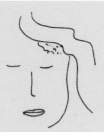

Psoriasis

Nutrition and herbal medicine considerations

Not all psoriasis is responsive to dietary change. Those I've seen respond to dietary changes have benefited from:

- Avoiding pork and tomatoes for a trial period of four weeks.

- If that doesn't work, trial dairy-free for four weeks as some cases of psoriasis begin during or after a strep infection.

- EFA supplementation.

- Supplementing zinc.

Emotions or beliefs to explore

- Enquire within if you (subconsciously) decided to 'thicken your skin' to avoid emotional hurts.

- Is there some sort of separation conflict related to a family member, friend, home, or pet? (1)

- Trying to please too many people who you perceive are authorities (1).

- Feeling overwhelmed.

- Perfectionism.

Rosacea

Nutrition and herbal medicine considerations

- Support the liver (refer to page 91 for considerations about how to do this).

- Follow a strict dairy-free diet trial for a minimum of four weeks—you will notice significantly less redness by the end of this trial period if you are going to respond.

- EFAs can also be highly beneficial.

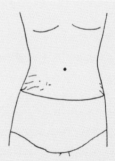

Scars and stretch marks

Nutrition and herbal medicine considerations

- Consider taking additional vitamin C.

- Zinc supplementation is almost always needed.

- Using lavender oil and/or calendula oil can also be beneficial to decreasing the appearance of scars.

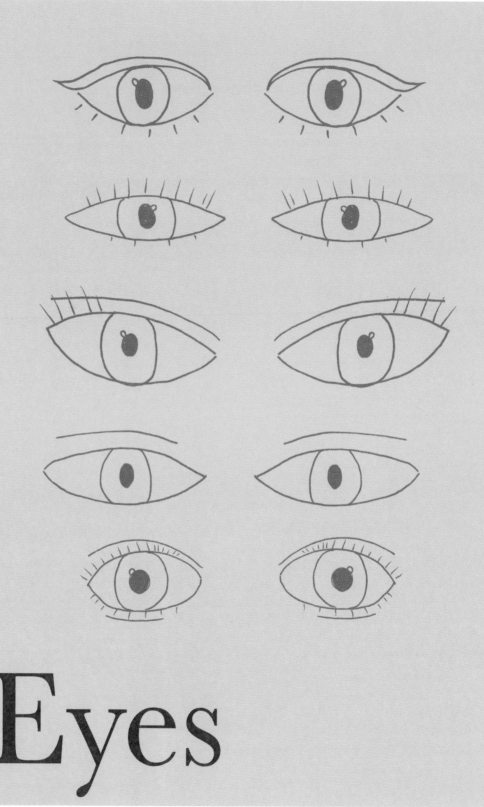

Eyes

Dr Libby Weaver

Dark circles

Nutrition and herbal medicine considerations

- Focus on digestion and/or liver support.

- Based on what you have learnt in this book and what has welled up for you, trial either a dairy-free diet or a gluten-free diet for four weeks to see if it makes a difference. I have seen both dietary trials resolve dark circles, and I don't say that lightly.

- Liver herbs can also be beneficial.

Floaters in vision

Nutrition and herbal medicine considerations

- Focus on liver support.
- Check for iron deficiency.

Puffy eyes

Nutrition and herbal medicine considerations

- Adrenal support is very important.

- Switch to drinking only water or herbal tea for two weeks and see if this makes a difference.

Thinning outer third of eyebrow

Nutrition and herbal medicine considerations

- You need endocrine system support (remember, the pituitary gland is the mother gland).

- Focus particularly on thyroid support.

- You may even like to have some thyroid tests done. However, remember that if they show up in the 'normal' range they may be skewed one way, and in this case, you need to work with a holistic health professional (integrative GP, highly experienced, degree-qualified naturopath or holistic nutritionist) to treat the signs that your body is giving you, rather than just the blood results.

Emotions or beliefs to explore

- What do you, as an individual, require to feel 'safe'?

- When is it going to be my turn?

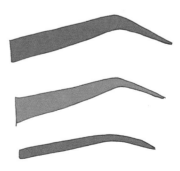

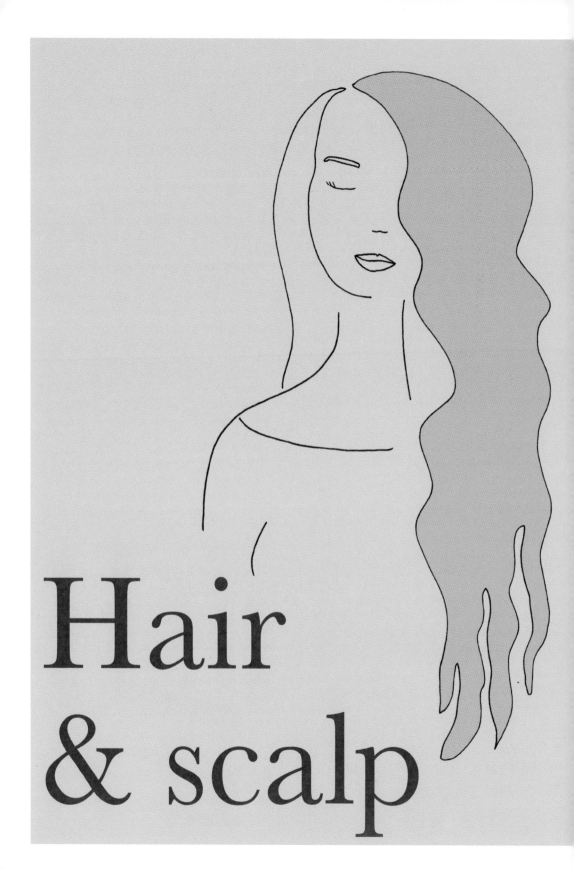

Hair
& scalp

Dr Libby Weaver

Brittle hair

Nutrition and herbal medicine considerations

Support your:

- Thyroid.
- Adrenals.

Useful nutrients include:

- EFAs.
- Vitamin C.

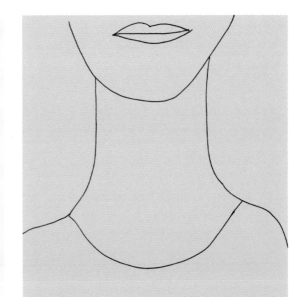

Grey hair

Nutrition and herbal medicine considerations

Head hair going grey is mostly genetic and hereditary. However, TCM treats grey hair by using herbs to support the kidneys.

I have only known people of Asian heritage who have used these herbs, but that is not to say they won't benefit people of non-Asian heritage. If pubic hairs start to go grey, it can be a sign that adrenal support is necessary.

Emotions or beliefs to explore

- If your hair went grey prematurely (your parents went grey much later than you), consider issues that may have shocked you or initiated worry or sorrow (1).

Hairy chin, facial hair

Nutrition and herbal medicine considerations

This is often due to increased levels of androgens in the skin. Start with stress hormone management strategies, including the restorative practices discussed throughout the book.

When facial hair has started to occur, it is very important for these girls/women to learn how to live from a calm place, not just access a calm place when they do yoga and then go back to living with adrenal-depleting intensity.

Paeonia and licorice as a herbal combination can also assist with this.

Dandruff, flaky scalp

Nutrition and herbal medicine considerations

This could be linked to a vitamin A deficiency, EFA deficiency, or gut dysbiosis. If you believe that for you it is more likely to be the latter, and that there are some less-than-friendly bacterial species living in your large intestine, trial a diet where you eat zero refined sugar and only whole food sources of carbs, such as root vegetables, brown rice and quinoa. Trial this initially for four weeks and, if you feel there is an improvement, continue for a total of three months to assess if it will resolve in this period. You might also like to add more coconut to your diet, as the lauric acid may also assist the scalp. Amp up the greens and the whole food fat in your diet as well. Apple cider vinegar before meals can also help via its stimulation of stomach acid.

Some hair experts suggest not washing your hair and, if you have access to it, swimming in the ocean each day instead.

Emotions or beliefs to explore

- Are you rushing and attempting to get too much done? (1)

- You have a tendency to behave with urgency, even when it's not necessary and/or set unrealistic deadlines (1).

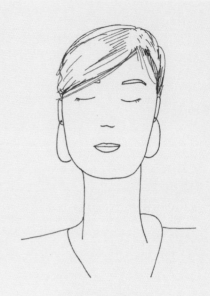

Hair loss

Nutrition and herbal medicine considerations

Support your:

- Thyroid.
- Adrenals.
- Sex hormone balance.

Consider if you are deficient in:

- Vitamin D.
- Zinc.
- Iron.
- Iodine.

Emotions or beliefs to explore

- Difficulty expressing feelings—fearing and avoiding conflicts (1); in my experience with patients, this is often (but not always) with a family member.

- Trust, control issues (1).

- Major stress or relationship conflict (1).

"

AS IF YOU WERE ON FIRE FROM WITHIN.

THE MOON LIVES IN THE LINING OF YOUR SKIN.

"

— Pablo Neruda

Lips

Dr Libby Weaver

Lips and around the mouth

Bad breath

Nutrition and herbal medicine considerations

- Focus on resolving gut/digestion challenges.

Emotions or beliefs to explore

- Anger and revenge thoughts (2).
- Unrealistic expectations on self or others in unrealistic time frames (1).
- Pressure—nothing is happening as fast as you want it to (1).

Chapped lips

Nutrition and herbal medicine considerations

- Focus on digestive system support, and support stomach acid production using lemon juice in warm water or apple cider vinegar.

Teeth strength and prevention of cavities

Nutrition and herbal medicine considerations

The teeth-strengthening minerals include:

- Calcium.
- Magnesium.
- Manganese.
- Boron.
- Vitamin D.

If you notice significant changes to your teeth, consider:

- Seeing a holistic dentist.
- Focus on a refined sugar-free, mineral-rich way of eating.
- Explore the need for adrenal support.
- Brush twice daily.
- Smile.

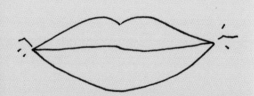

Cracks at the corners of the mouth

Nutrition and herbal medicine considerations

- These can be due to a vitamin B deficiency, an iron deficiency, or both.

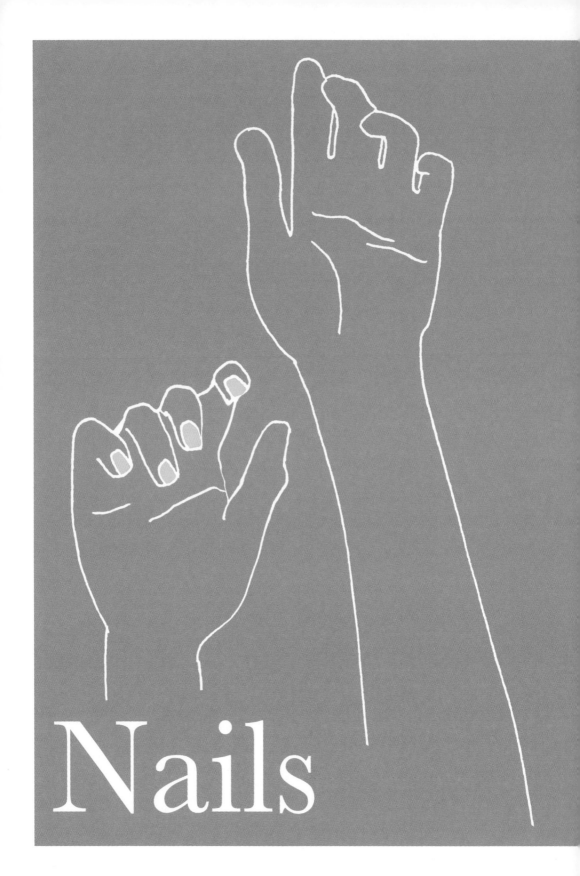

Nails

Dr Libby Weaver

Dull nails

Nutrition and herbal medicine considerations

This can indicate:

- A poor-quality diet and a greater need for nutrients.
- Poor digestion.
- Inadequate dietary protein consumption or poor digestion of protein (try supporting stomach acid production with apple cider vinegar if this is suspected).
- Iron deficiency.
- Folate deficiency (less common).

Eat more whole real food, and focus on supporting digestion.

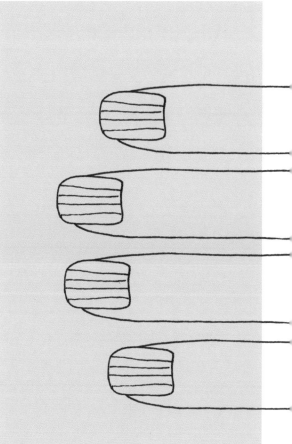

Lined nails (grooves across the nail)

Nutrition and herbal medicine considerations

- Inadequate dietary protein consumption or poor digestion of protein (try supporting stomach acid production with apple cider vinegar if this is suspected).
- Adrenal support may be needed, and restorative practices are essential.

Lined nails (grooves from base to tip)

Nutrition and herbal medicine considerations

- This can indicate a mineral deficiency, such as calcium and magnesium.
- It can also indicate that the thyroid needs support.

Pale, brittle, withered or weak nails

Nutrition and herbal medicine considerations

- Liver support is usually necessary.

- It can also indicate an iron deficiency. If dietary iron intake is good, have iron blood studies done to determine if a deficiency exists. If so, explore why. 'Unexplained' iron deficiency can highlight digestive system challenges or it can be a sign of undiagnosed coeliac disease.

Soft nails

Nutrition and herbal medicine considerations

- Make sure you are getting adequate dietary protein. To make keratin, a tough protein that is a major component in hard, strong nails, the body needs high-quality protein.

- If you are sure that you are, focus on digestive system support.

Peeling or scabby cuticles

Nutrition and herbal medicine considerations

- This can be due to EFA deficiency.

- Do you pick your nails or around your nails? Apply some calming strategies you learnt throughout the book as this is a common behaviour if people feel quite anxious.

- Try rubbing a little coconut oil or face oil around your nail beds each evening. Or keep a face oil on your desk to rub into your nails across the day, if you pick your nails at work.

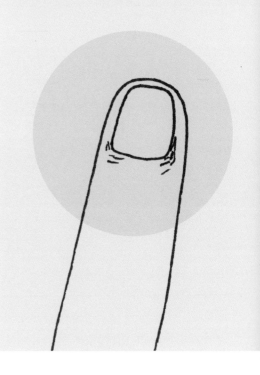

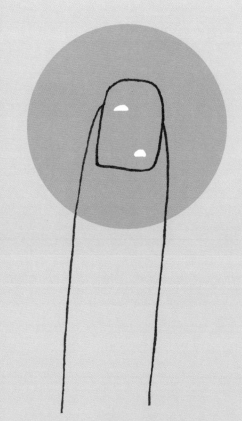

Spoon-shaped nails

Nutrition and herbal medicine considerations

- This is often due to iron deficiency.

- May also be the result of deficiencies in vitamin B12 and/ or folate.

- If you see your nails develop into a spoon shape, please see your GP for blood tests for the above nutrients.

Above all else, care so deeply for your dear self that you want to nourish yourself well with nutrient-dense foods, periods of rest, kind and curious thoughts (as opposed to harsh and judgemental) and practices that support your own individual wellbeing.

Don't make these things extras on your to-do list. See your opportunity to care for yourself as a tremendously special gift. See your body as a miracle doing her best to give you the most amazing quality of life. Support her in her mission to give you such an extraordinary gift through the choices you make, the thoughts you think and the actions you take.

White spots on nails

Nutrition and herbal medicine considerations

- This can indicate a zinc deficiency, but not always.

- It can be a sign that the nail beds were injured during a manicure (or something else).

- May be a reaction to a new nail polish.

- Nails reacting to cleaning products (try wearing gloves to see if it resolves).

"
Everything in the universe is a pitcher brimming with wisdom and beauty.
"

— Rumi

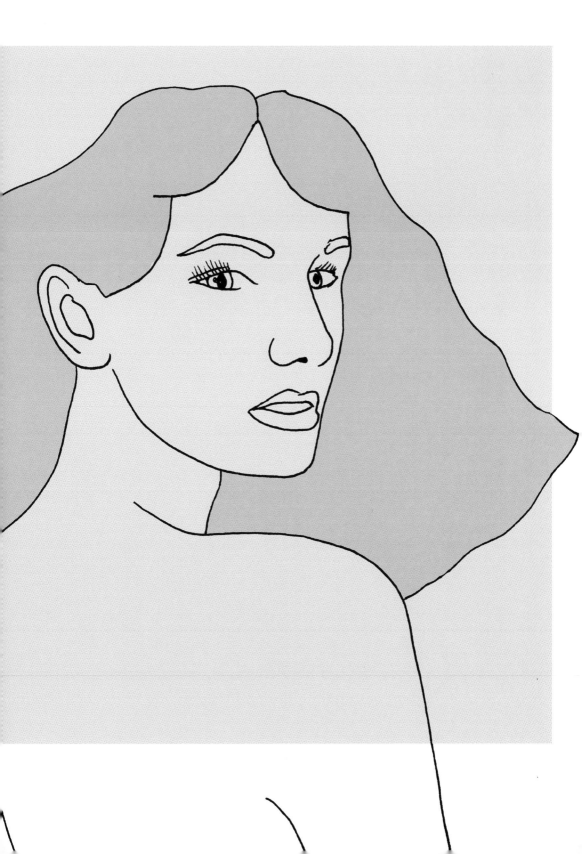

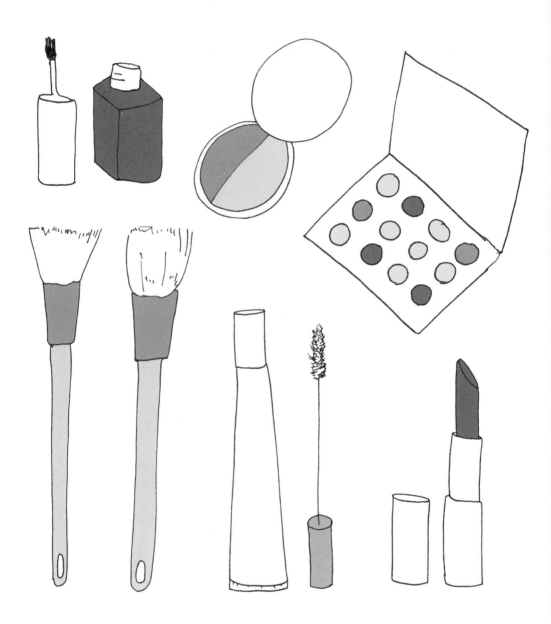

Dr Libby Weaver

On the surface

Substances to carefully consider

———

What we put on our skin matters. So often when we buy a new moisturising cream that feels and smells luxurious we don't pause to consider that whatever is in that product will be absorbed into our bloodstream—with the potential to either enhance our inner health or demand even more of our (potentially) already overloaded biochemical pathways of detoxification. When we get sunburn, we're encouraged to rub aloe vera over the affected area because it helps to soothe it. Do you think it does this just by sitting on the top of the skin? Of course not. It is the absorption of the substances in the aloe vera through the skin that provide the skin with substances it needs to repair and counteract the effects of the sun damage. Or perhaps you've used a topical hormone cream or a nicotine patch—other examples that highlight how we absorb things through our skin. What we put on our skin matters. We don't always look critically at the ingredients in a product because we assume that because it's on the shelf it must be safe for us to use.

Research is continuing into the detrimental effects of certain ingredients that have made their way into everything from food, to skincare products, to what we clean our homes with. The growing body of knowledge in this area only seeks to support better human and planetary health as we become aware of some of the longer term consequences of our exposure to these substances.

It is important to understand that dose is everything when it comes to 'toxins'. For example, the body needs iodine to function—to survive—and an adult female needs 150 micrograms per day to meet these basic requirements. Yet if someone consumed 150 grams of iodine, it would be toxic to them; it could poison them. Literally. There is no question that we are now exposed to more pollutants than ever before via what we eat, drink, inhale and put on our skin.

Without taking the lid completely off that box, simply consider that there are more cars on the road than ever before. My point is, there are some exposures we can control—we can change the skincare products we use to ones that don't contain any concerning ingredients so that fewer potentially problematic substances go in—while there are numerous environmental exposures that we have very little, if any, control over.

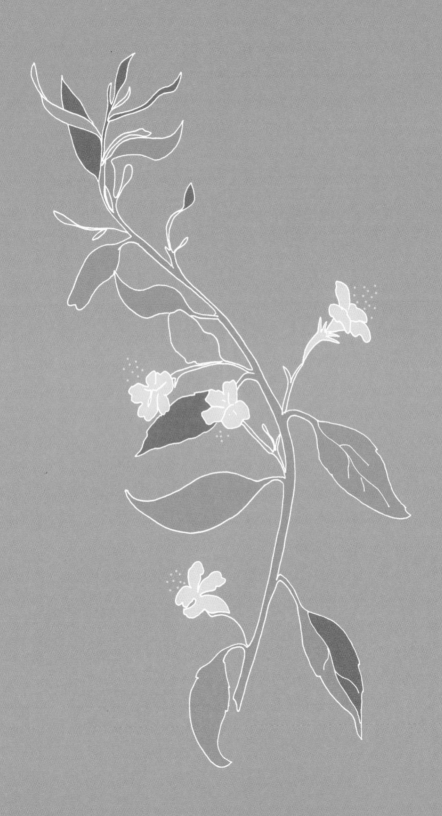

Dr Libby Weaver

Again, think about cars on the road. So, my focus is to encourage you to minimise your exposures where you can and support your body's detoxification and elimination pathways to excrete what you are exposed to that enters your body. For it is only when they remain in your tissues that any of these substances can be a problem.

Having said that, consider also that anything you put down the kitchen sink as well as the water from your shower or when you flush the toilet—the contents of your urine, faeces and cleaning products—all end up in some water or waterway somewhere. Some of these have their own ecosystems and support the life of aquatic creatures, and form part of your food chain and the food chain of other species.

I was reminded of this very powerfully when I was doing my PhD. Another PhD candidate, who was a marine biologist, originally set out in his research to look at aspects of oyster health. Part of his work involved taking water samples from four different areas where oysters are grown to see if substances (predominantly nutrients) in the water might be impacting what was occurring with the oysters. That part of his project was waylaid, however, as what he was finding in the water was too shocking not to investigate it further.

Of the substances being found, the two in the highest concentration were penicillin (from antibiotics) and a synthetic form of estrogen, found only in estrogen-based medications (not the estrogen the body makes) such as that found in hormone replacement therapy (HRT) and the OCP.

Nothing we do has zero effect. Everything creates a ripple. So, we need to decide on the type of ripple we want to make.

With that in mind, let's explore some of the ingredients that have a growing body of research behind them that shows they are of some concern to human health and/or the health of aquatic environments. Then we'll look at what you might like to use instead, in the simplification of your 'beauty' routine.

SKINCARE INGREDIENTS TO BE MINDFUL OF

Some of the skincare ingredients you want to be conscious of being exposed to and reduce your exposure to include:

- butylated hydroxyanisole (BHA) and butylated hydroxytoluene (BHT)
- parabens
- sodium laureth sulfate, also referred to as sodium lauryl ether sulfate (SLES)
- phthalates, such as dibutyl phthalate
- resorcinol
- diethanolamine (DEA) and DEA compounds
- polyethylene glycols (PEGs)
- formaldehyde-releasing agents
- triclosan
- petrolatum
- siloxanes.

Let's examine a few in more detail so you can see where some of the health concerns lie.

BHA AND BHT

- are synthetic antioxidants used as preservatives in a range of cosmetics, including moisturisers and lipsticks (1)

- have been shown that they can induce allergic reactions in the skin (2).

BHA:

- has been classified as a 'possible human carcinogen' by The International Agency for Research on Cancer (3)

- is listed as a Category 1 priority substance by The European Commission on Endocrine Disruption, based on evidence that it interferes with hormone function (4). The concern with the latter is the potential consequences on the endocrine system and on the body's ability to regulate and balance sex hormones.

PARABENS

- are preservatives used in many cosmetic and personal care products

- are used as ingredients in fragrances, but this isn't usually listed on the label

- can penetrate the skin (5)

- are listed as Category 1 priority substances by The European Commission on Endocrine Disruption, based on evidence that they interfere with hormone function (6)

- can mimic estrogen and have been detected in human breast cancer tissues (7)

- have been shown to react with UVB when applied to the skin, which leads to accelerated skin ageing and DNA damage (8).

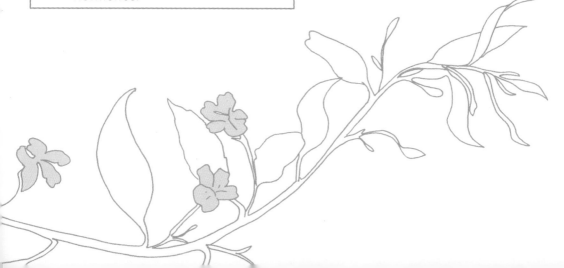

SLES

Sodium laureth sulfate/sodium lauryl ether sulfate:

- is used primarily as a detergent in cosmetics
- makes products bubble and foam
- is commonly found in shampoos, facial cleansers and shower gels
- may be contaminated with measurable amounts of ethylene oxide and 1,4-dioxane, depending on how it is manufactured (9).

Ethylene oxide:

- is a 'known human carcinogen', according to The International Agency for Research on Cancer (10)
- can harm the nervous system (11)
- is classified as a possible developmental toxicant based on evidence that it may interfere with human development, according to the California Environmental Protection Agency (12).

1,4-dioxane:

- is referred to as a substance 'reasonably considered to be a human carcinogen' by The International Agency for Research on Cancer (13)
- is persistent, which means it doesn't easily break down and can remain in the environment long after it goes down the drain (14).

RESORCINOL

- is used as an antiseptic and disinfectant
- found in topical treatments for acne, eczema, psoriasis, seborrhoeic dermatitis, warts and corns
- is found in hair dyes
- has been linked with thyroid dysfunction (15).

DEA

and DEA compounds such as cocamide and lauramide DEA:

- are used to make cosmetics creamy or sudsy
- are mainly found in moisturisers, sunscreens, soaps, cleansers and shampoos
- have been shown to cause liver cancers and precancerous changes in the skin and thyroid, with high-dose exposures in laboratory experiments over two years (16)
- are classified as 'hazardous' to the environment due to their 'acute toxicity to aquatic organisms and potential for bioaccumulation' by the Danish Environmental Protection Agency (17).

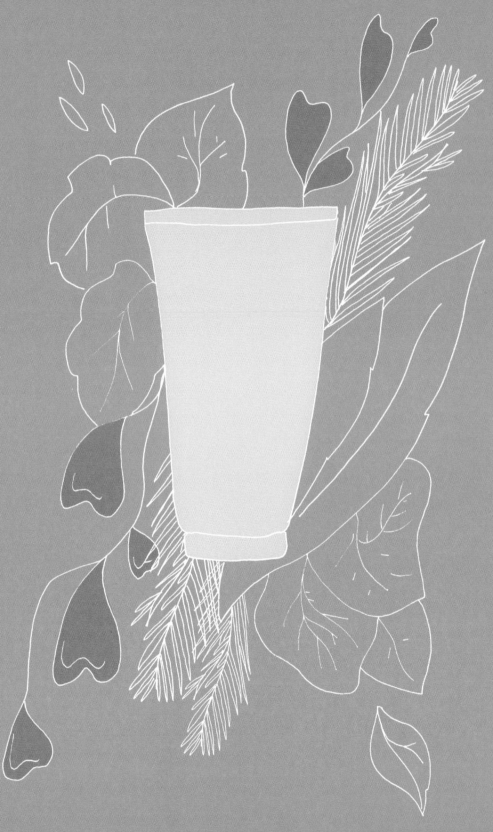

Dr Libby Weaver

In summary, you might decide it is a good idea to start to transition to less synthetic skincare. For example, when your lipstick, mascara or foundation next runs out, consider replacing them with a brand that doesn't contain any of the ingredients just discussed. Small steps can have an enormous payback to you and the planet in the long term. As well as the aforementioned ingredients, try looking for products that are free from synthetic fragrances, colours, preservatives, animal derivatives and petrochemicals.

THERE ARE MANY EFFECTIVE SKINCARE RANGES THAT DON'T CONTAIN ANY OF THE INGREDIENTS MENTIONED ABOVE. SEEK THEM OUT.

Or you might like to make your own. You can make your own oil-based cleanser and moisturiser, for example. You can make a toner using witch hazel as a base and you have your basic three face needs. Do what is practical for you and gradually transition what you use on your miraculous body. Ultimately, choose skincare that supports the function of your skin, and personal care products that support your overall health as well as that of the planet, rather than those that risk disrupting these precious ecosystems.

FEMININE HYGIENE PRODUCTS

Another consideration in minimising your exposure to problematic substances and a major environmental concern relates to the types of feminine hygiene products you use. Pads, and tampons in particular, as they enter the body, rest incredibly close to parts of you that need the utmost care. A tampon is positioned inside the vagina, just below the cervix while in your body. In the same way you absorb substances through the skin on the outside of your body, substances (in tampons) can be absorbed by the vaginal mucosa from where they pass almost directly into your bloodstream.

One of the main ingredients in a tampon is cotton and, although steps are being taken to reduce the amount of pesticides being used to spray cotton worldwide, it is still a crop with that requires relatively intensive pesticide use. In a number of countries where cotton is grown, it appears in the top four of the most sprayed crops. The top four usually contain cotton, soy, maize and 'cereals' in general (18). Other ingredients typically found in or used in the production of conventional feminine hygiene products include:

- plastics, which can take hundreds of years to degrade if they end up in landfill or if they make their way into our marine environments, damaging these ecosystems and making their way into our food chain and the food chain of other species. We are yet to truly understand the implications of having plastics inside our body. Some may be harmless. Some may not be. We don't know yet. I, for one, am not prepared to be a guinea pig. Regardless of whether you use conventional or organic feminine hygiene products, please don't ever flush a tampon down the toilet.

- **chlorine bleach**, of which dioxin is a by-product. Dioxin is an organochlorine, known to disrupt the endocrine and reproductive systems in both humans and animals (19). It is also categorised as 'highly toxic' and a 'known human carcinogen' by the World Health Organization (WHO) (20). According to WHO, 'once dioxins enter the body, they last a long time because of their chemical stability and their ability to be absorbed by fat tissue, where they are then stored in the body. Their half-life in the body is estimated to be 7 to 11 years.' (20). A report in *Time* magazine in 2016 (21), discussed research conducted by a professor of microbiology and pathology who stated that 'the amount of dioxin in tampons is low today compared to when manufacturers used different bleaching methods. But it is still present, and its effect is cumulative.' And most women use them across their entire reproductive years, which might be 40 years or more.

- **fragrance**, which can increase our exposure to phthalates (22), which as you learnt above, are a class of suspected endocrine disruptors.

It has been estimated that Western women use between 9,000 and 12,000 tampons (and/or pads) over a lifetime, based on the following calculation:

1 tampon every 4 hours = 4 tampons per day (if you use a pad overnight).

If you menstruate for 5 days (periods are typically 3 to 7 days in length), this is 4 tampons per day x 5 days of bleeding = 20 tampons per menstrual cycle.

If you menstruate from the age of 12 to the age of 54 this is 42 years which means, without a pregnancy, you'd have 504 periods or 2,520 days of menstruation.

IF YOU USE 4 TAMPONS PER DAY, 4 X 2,520 DAYS = 10,080 TAMPONS USED ACROSS YOUR LIFE.

Given these statistics and all they offer us to consider, it may be wise to explore what feminine care products you use, both for you and the planet. Here are some options.

- Choose non-fragranced products.

- Look for products from companies who list their ingredients on the label and are transparent about what they put into their tampons. Labelling of feminine hygiene products is not necessary by law so seek out those who are proud of what they include, as well as what they leave out.

- Choose only certified organic pads and tampons for your health and that of the environment. A number of companies in many Western countries, with a great ethos based on caring for women's health as well as the planet's, have created a range of feminine care products, some of which are available in supermarkets, making it so easy for you to include these in your regular shop. Seek them out where you live!

- Explore using a menstrual cup, which is usually made from silicone and is inserted into the vagina to catch the menstrual blood. It sits lower down than a tampon and after four to eight hours you simply remove it, and empty the blood into the toilet. It is best to have at least two of them so you can sterilise the one you've just used in very hot water and reinsert the clean, dry one.

Make a choice based on what is comfortable for you, given what you now understand, a choice that takes such good care of three precious ecosystems: your reproductive system, your general health and our environment.

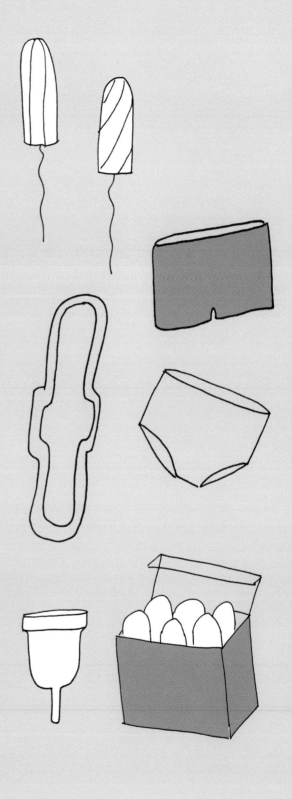

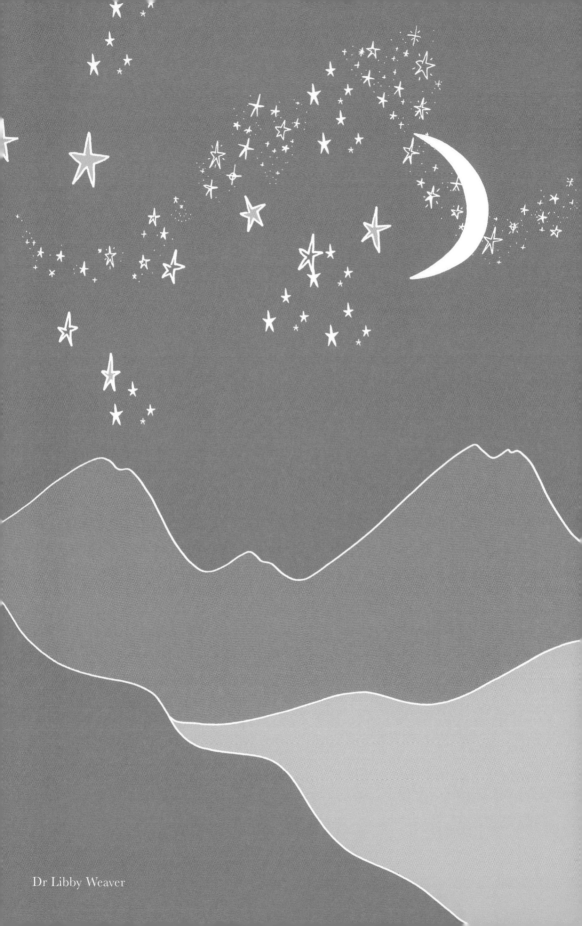

Dr Libby Weaver

Courageously beautiful

Getting back in touch with your true essence

Trust is the opposite of stress and, therefore, trust is one of the most impactful traits that you can embrace for your beauty and, of course, for your quality of life. The relaxation and relief of tension that is visible in your face and posture, the less relentless stress hormone production and the biochemical and nutritional benefits this brings to your beauty bits, the mental and emotional peace it offers—trust is the ultimate beauty elixir.

As the Serenity Prayer (1) suggests, there are things that require us to act courageously to change things in our lives or in the world, situations we might care about but don't like, or that are unacceptable to us. Yet there are also things that we can't change, perhaps just at the moment or perhaps longer term—you can't really know that yet (another opportunity for trust)—and in accepting this, you can find a whole slice of inner peace. We need to cultivate wisdom to be able to feel into the difference between stepping up and out against what needs changing and what just is what it is. For when you fight with what is, you suffer. It is curious that so many people seek joy when they themselves are the source of it.

We have a tendency to see things in the world, including traits in ourselves, as polar opposites. Good or bad. Right or wrong. Love or hate. Yet between the poles can be shades of other emotions when we allow ourselves to not stick to the extremes. Not to mention that we would lack appreciation of one without the other. For example, light without darkness could not be appreciated for its radiance. Pleasure without even a smidgen of pain can't really be truly sweet. Opposites provide relevance and enhance each other. So, when you judge yourself to be one, often harsh thing, you miss so many of the other parts that also make you beautiful.

When do you learn most? When you are happy and content or when you are suffering and feel like things have fallen apart? Almost always it's the latter. It is through our pain that we have the opportunity to grow. Which is why I suggest throughout the book that there is no such thing as failure, there is only feedback. For when we perceive that we have failed—at work, school, university, in a relationship, within our body—immense wisdom is on offer. And this fosters our growth and ability to contribute back to the world. Compassion springs forth from experiencing heartache, for example.

So rather than allow some of the tougher experiences in life to diminish your inner light, remember to value the polarities as well as the shades and never forget that life truly does happen for you. Trust that everything occurs or does not occur in alignment with the divine unfolding of your incredibly special and unique life. Embrace a sense of humour so that you can more easily choose lightness in your approach to things over weightiness, and so that you may move swiftly through any pain, rather than have it be debilitating.

Do your best to approach each day with a feeling of wonder and gratitude—for what surrounds you and what is within you. By enhancing your connection to your inner life, you live in touch with your own beauty and it shines out of your eyes, lighting up the lives of those you share time and space with.

I CANNOT ENCOURAGE YOU ENOUGH TO SPEND TIME IN NATURE.

This strengthens that inner connection as the rhythms of Nature offer calmness, clarity and remind you to trust yourself. Nature is not only an immense source of external beauty, but also a nurturing force that can restore physical and emotional health and beauty. Spend time in Nature observing, and feeling grateful, letting Nature's grace wash over you.

Remember that beauty is a light in your soul. It is in everyone. It's just that at some point, we tend to stop believing in our own preciousness, our own beauty. Yet as I asked you to consider throughout the book, do you stop believing in the sun just because the moon has come out? Your beauty may momentarily disappear from your own view, but it is always there. It just gets clouded over by behavioural patterns, challenging life experiences, beliefs based on what others have said (remembering that this is a reflection of what they believe about themselves, not about who you are), images and stories from the media and social media. You just need to explore what is obstructing your view. Your beauty is always present, yearning for you to believe in yourself again. You were born believing in yourself and the gold within. You just forget sometimes. But I want to encourage you with all of my heart to awaken that part of you that might have gone to sleep.

Take such good care of you, including via how you nourish yourself and through the thoughts you think. Become so awake to how you tell yourself you have to be to be loved or liked or to fit in. For you just need to be your beautiful, authentic self. Trust yourself, for as soon as you trust yourself again, you will know how to live (2). And the radiance that shines from that authentic, soul-guided way of living lights up the whole sky.

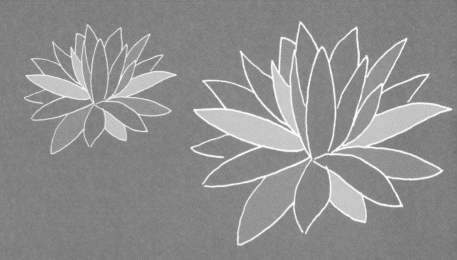

Do your best to approach each day with

A FEELING
OF WONDER
AND
GRATITUDE

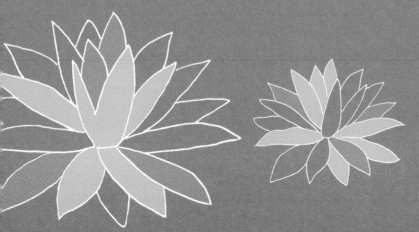

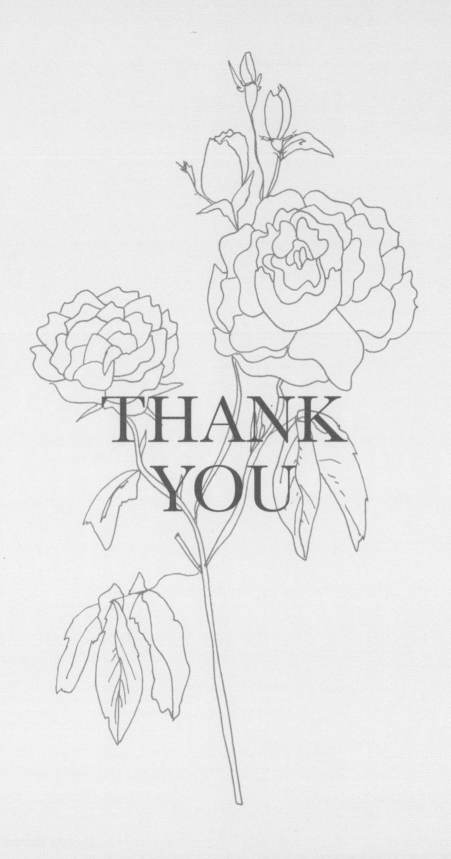

THANK
YOU

Acknowledgments

Work is play when you love what you do and love who you "work" with. Biggest heartfelt thanks to Sarah, my editor. Not only are you immensely gifted with words but your heart knows my brain and heart and I thank you deeply for both. Thank you Maddy for your enthusiasm, ideas and insights and all that you contribute every day. To Bree, thank you for your care and attention to detail. Thank you to Chris for knowing this book needed to be born and your encouragement to bring it to life. And to Karl for the gifts of my ongoing Karlucation while I wrote this book. Biggest neon lit up sign thanks to Steph for the beautiful illustrations and design of this book. Your creativity knows no bounds and I am so grateful to you for sharing your gifts on these pages. With love and thanks to you all.

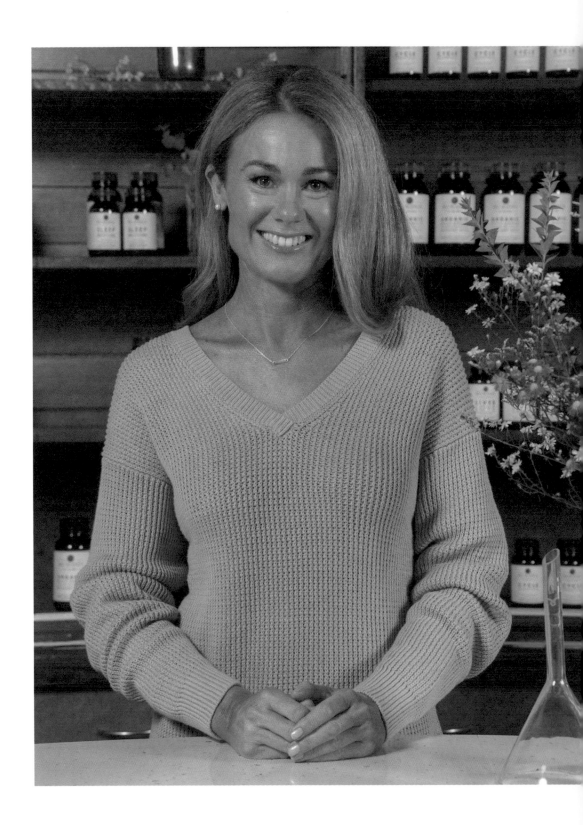

Dr Libby Weaver

About Dr Libby

Nutritional biochemist, author and speaker

———

Dr Libby Weaver (PhD) is one of Australasia's leading nutritional biochemists, an author, a speaker and founder of the food-based supplement range, Bio Blends.

Armed with an abundance of knowledge, scientific research and a true desire to help people regain their energy and vitality, Dr Libby empowers and inspires people to take charge of their health and happiness through her books, live events and nutritional support range.

Having sold over 350,000 books across New Zealand and Australia, she is a eleven-times bestselling author.

A respected international speaker, Dr Libby's expertise in nutritional biochemistry has led her to share the stage with Marianne Williamson, Sir Richard Branson, Tony Robbins and Dr Oz. She is regularly called on as an authoritative figure in the health and wellness industry and has been featured in numerous media publications including *The Times, The Huffington Post, Sydney Morning Herald, the Australian Women's Weekly* and she appears regularly on breakfast radio and television.

With a natural ability to break even the most complex of concepts into layperson's terms, Dr Libby's health messages embrace her unique three-pillared approach that explores the interplay between nutrition, emotions and the biochemistry of the body.

It's no surprise that when it comes to achieving and maintaining ultimate health and wellbeing, Hollywood stars Deborra-lee Furness and Hugh Jackman describe her as a 'one stop shop in achieving and maintaining ultimate health and wellbeing.'

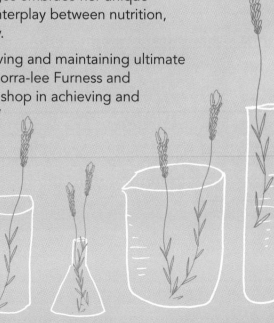

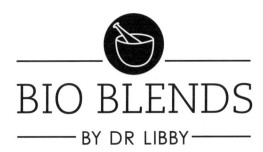

BIO BLENDS

— BY DR LIBBY —

food-based supplements

Most supplements are made in a lab using synthetic ingredients, whereas Bio Blends supplements are entirely food-based. This means they are made only from food, plants and herbs; substances your body knows what to do with. Dr Libby scoured the world to find the highest quality ingredients and, using her twenty years of experience, formulated these products to help your body experience exceptional health.

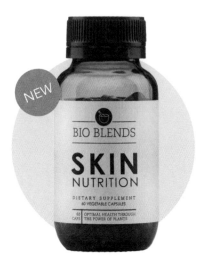

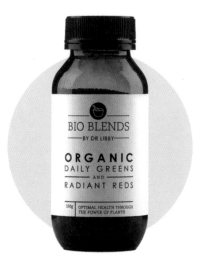

Skin Nutrition

A nutrient-rich formula with a combination of healing plants that work to improve skin radiance and tone, reduce redness and increase blood circulation—think better nutrient delivery to the skin. Learn more over the page.

Organic Daily Greens & Radiant Reds

Precisely formulated to contain a powerhouse of antioxidants, substances that help to combat premature ageing. This delicious powder can be enjoyed daily in water or your favourite smoothie.

Find out more at www.bioblends.co.nz

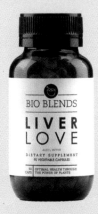

Liver Love

Supports liver regeneration and detoxification and assists your liver to process the harmful liver loaders that could be contributing to your headaches, gut problems, such as bloating and constipation, irritability, fatigue, congested skin, and unexplained increases in body fat.

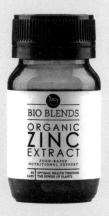

Organic Zinc

Zinc is involved in over 300 processes inside your body and most people today aren't getting enough of it. This superstar nutrient works with your body to help you have a healthy immune system, experience great energy, achieve optimal digestion and have radiant hair, skin and eyes.

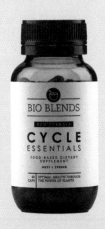

Cycle Essentials

A potent blend of foods, plants and herbs which promote healthy progesterone production and help you address PMS, period pain, bloating, sugar cravings and mood fluctuations, leading to a period that simply shows up.

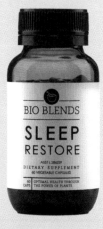

Sleep Restore

The potent combination of herbs has a calming action on our nervous system, easing anxious feelings and most importantly helping to uncoil a busy mind to support short-term through to long-term sleep challenges, including insomnia.

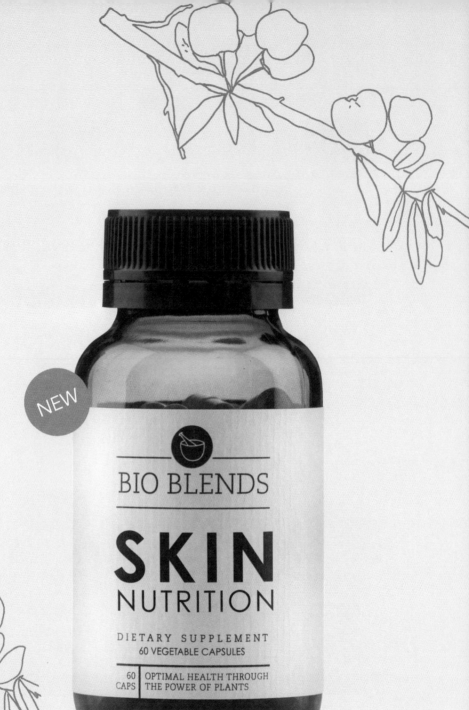

NEW

BIO BLENDS

SKIN
NUTRITION

DIETARY SUPPLEMENT
60 VEGETABLE CAPSULES

60
CAPS

OPTIMAL HEALTH THROUGH
THE POWER OF PLANTS

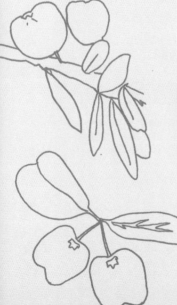

Skin Nutrition

Beauty really is an inside job.

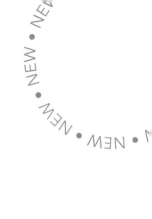

Do you feel like your skin looks stressed out and tired? Or are you often frustrated by skin concerns such as acne, dark circles, cellulite, uneven skin tone, dryness, stretch marks, rosacea or signs of ageing? Then your skin may need more nutrients in order to heal from the inside out.

Skin Nutrition is an antioxidant-rich formula that combines the healing benefits of grape seed, melon extract, gotu kola, guava leaf extract and acerola berries to give your skin what it needs to radiate with health.

Working with the body, this formulation has been proven to reduce redness and spots, provide relief from dark circles under the eye, improve collagen stability and increase circulation (think better nutrient delivery to the skin) (1).

In fact, women aged between 40 and 70 years who trialled this formulation experienced an increase in both luminosity and the elasticity of their skin, in just two months (1).

Made entirely from food, Skin Nutrition is highly bioavailable as it only contains nutrients found in nature.

SKIN NUTRITION WORKS TO:

- Improve skin radiance
- Provide antioxidant protection, which helps to prevent skin cell damage
- Improve blood circulation to fully oxygenate, nourish and hydrate the skin
- Optimise skin colour and reduce pigmentation spots
- Protect skin fibres to preserve elasticity and suppleness
- Decrease dark circles under the eyes

Nourish your skin with the nutrients it needs for a clear and luminous complexion. For best results take for two to three months, or as long as you are appreciating the benefits.

1. Dumoulin, M. Gaudout, D. and Lemaire, B. (2016) "Clinical effects of an oral supplement rich in antioxidants on skin radiance in women" Clinical, Cosmetic and Investigational Dermatology. 9:315–324.

ALSO BY DR LIBBY WEAVER

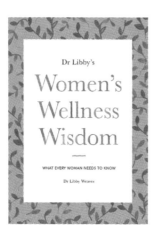

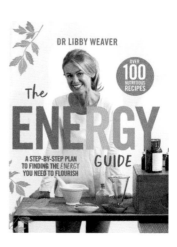

Women's Wellness Wisdom

A definitive guidebook for women, *Women's Wellness Wisdom* includes beautiful imagery, step-by-step guides, worksheets and real-life examples, helping you uncover the sources of your challenges and empowering you with the knowledge to better understand your body. Learn what women of all ages need to know from this inspiring book.

The Energy Guide

Authoritative and compassionate, *The Energy Guide,* which includes over 100 recipes and meal ideas, will help you to reboot your diet, improve your sleep, understand your hormones, reduce your stress and transform the way you think about your energy and your wellbeing.

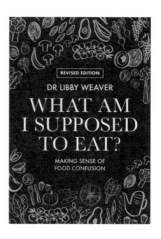

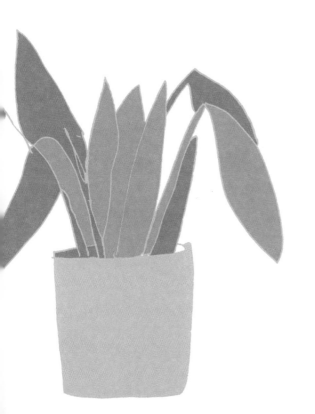

What am I Supposed to Eat?

For many people, deciding what to eat is often filled with confusion, fuelled by temptation or convenience and leaves them begging the question, "So, what am I supposed to eat?" This book is a fork in the road when it comes to better understanding your food, your body, your appetite, your emotions and what is best for you to eat.

ALSO BY DR LIBBY WEAVER

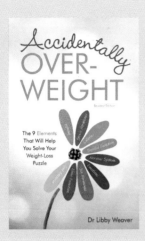

Accidentally Overweight

Accidentally Overweight explores the must-know nine factors essential to successful and sustainable weight loss. They include stress hormones, sex hormones, thyroid function and gut bacteria.

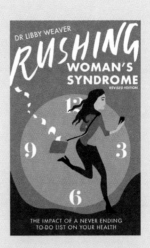

Rushing Woman's Syndrome

Rushing Woman's Syndrome offers you real solutions to both the biochemistry and the emotional patterns of the rush. What you need to do in a day may not change but how you show up can revolutionise how you experience each day and how others experience you.

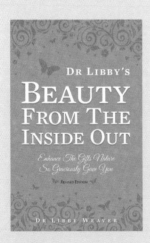

Beauty from the Inside Out

Beauty from the Inside Out is a must-have beauty book for women of all ages. Enjoy radiating your own unique sparkle from the inside out, and learn how everything from nutrients to emotions impacts what is displayed on the outside.

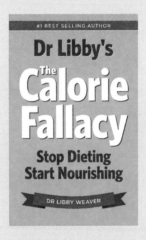

The Calorie Fallacy

This book arms you with the wisdom to stop dieting and depriving yourself and start thriving. Stop dieting and start nourishing and start living with a new freedom with your relationship with food and your body.

ALSO BY DR LIBBY WEAVER

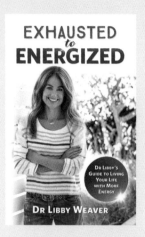

Exhausted to Energized

Everything in life is more difficult when we are exhausted. *Exhausted to Energized* offers you simple but powerful strategies to help liberate you from exhaustion and live a life with more energy.

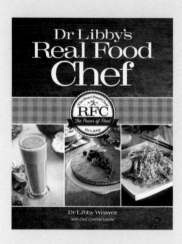

Real Food Chef

The *Real Food Chef* is a beautiful book that will revolutionise the way you are nourished. Filled with delicious and nutrient dense meals, drinks, snacks and sauces, this book educates and supports you to embrace a real food way of eating.

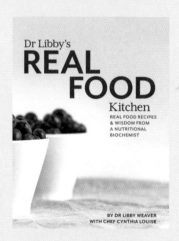

Real Food Kitchen

The *Real Food Kitchen* will inspire you to take better care of yourself with the delicious and nutritious recipes featured. Packed with even more nutritional information as well as recipes that are firm family favourites that have been 'real food chef-ified', you will love using this beautiful cookbook.

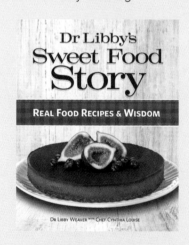

Sweet Food Story

Many people make great food choices for breakfast and lunch, and then at 3 o'clock in the afternoon they feel like someone else has taken over their body, their desire for sweet food can be so intense. The *Sweet Food Story* cookbook was created with this in mind, as a way of educating and supporting you to eat sweet food that serves your health.

References and Resources

I am regularly touched by the number of people who, after reading one of my books, write to me saying that it's like I've described their life or peeked at the pages of their journal. If, after reading *The Beauty Guide*, you would like to delve further into your physical or emotional health, I encourage you to check out my website where you will find all of my other book titles, weekend events, tours and courses.

If body fat or energy challenges are a daily battle for you, you might benefit from *Weight Loss for Women*, which is a nine-week practical online course overflowing with guidance and tuition to help you solve your weight loss puzzle.

Take a look at the blog too at:
www.drlibby.com

I also post health information each weekday on social media.

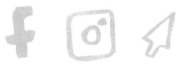

Connect with me there at:

www.facebook.com/DrLibbyLive
And on Instagram, find me as @drlibby

My passion is to educate and inspire, and to help people change the relationship they have with their bodies and their health and put the power of choice back in their hands. It is an honour to assist you in your optimal health journey.

I have cited some books and papers in this text and they are listed in full here if further reading in a particular area interests you.

Over the last 25 years I have read in excess of 10,000 books and research papers that have inspired and shaped my work. I have done my best to include those who have been instrumental in contributing to my work, as well as to this book.

There is additional referencing on my website: www.drlibby.com

REFERENCES AND RESOURCES

Understanding ageing

    1. http://learn.genetics.utah.edu/content/basics/telomeres/

The quality of your life

    1. Carver, C. (2017) *Soulful Simplicity*. New York City: Tarcherperigree.

Are you aggravated by acne?

    1. West Kurz, S. (2006) *Awakening Beauty*. New York City: Clarkson Potter Publishers.

Luscious locks

    1. Holmes, A., Blaxill, M. and Haley, B. (2003) "Reduced Levels of Mercury in First Baby Haircuts of Autistic Children" *International Journal of Toxicology*. 22 (4): 277-285.

    2. https://www.newscientist.com/article/dn3842-toxic-metal-clue-to-autism/

    3. https://www.gatewayworkshops.co.uk

    4. Food Standards Australia New Zealand. NUTTAB 2010 – Australian Food Composition Tables. Canberra, ACT.

    5. https://www.ncbi.nlm.nih.gov/pmc/articles/PMC2658806/

Nailing it

    1. https://courses.lumenlearning.com/boundless-ap/chapter/accessory-structures-of-the-skin/

Beauty wisdom

    1. http://sixdegreeshealth.ca/resources/facts-lists/healthy-blood/

    2. Serralach, O. (2018) *The Post-natal Depletion Cure.* New York City: goop press.

When things aren't what you want them to be

    1. Carver, C. (2017) *Soulful Simplicity*. New York City: Tarcherperigree.

    2. This is my interpretation of concepts I was first exposed to at live events by Dr John Demartini and Tony Robbins.

Lifting the veil on your values

    1. Demartini, J. (2013) *The Values Factor*. New York City: Penguin.

    2. https://drdemartini.com/value_determination

REFERENCES AND RESOURCES

Caring is beautiful

1. Rudy Francisco on twitter.com/rudyfranscisco posted on 20.12.2015

Culture of comparison

1. Chodron, P. (1996) *Awakening Loving-Kindness.* Boston: Shambhala Publications.

The pursuit of perfection

1. Robbins, T. (2009) *Date with Destiny* live event was where I first heard these questions asked.

Illumination

1. Williamson, M. (2009) *A Return To Love.* Sydney: Harper Collins.

Insights into beauty challenges

1. Demartini, J. (2016) *Prophecy II* workbooks from live event.
2. Hay, L. (2004) *You Can Heal Your Life.* Carlsbad: Hay House.

Beauty solutions

1. Demartini, J. (2016) *Prophecy II* workbooks from live event.
2. Hay, L. (2004) *You Can Heal Your Life.* Carlsbad: Hay House.
3. Dumoulin, M. Gaudout, D. and Lemaire, B. (2016) "Clinical effects of an oral supplement rich in antioxidants on skin radiance in women" *Clinical, Cosmetic and Investigational Dermatology.* 9:315–324.

On the surface

1. https://davidsuzuki.org/wp-content/uploads/2010/10/dirty-dozen-BACKGROUNDER.pdf
2. U.S. National Library of Medicine, in Haz-Map: Occupational Exposure to Hazardous Agents, 2010, http://hazmap.nlm.nih.gov. cited in https://davidsuzuki.org/queen-of-green/dirty-dozen-bha-bht/
3. IARC Monographs on the Evaluation of Carcinogenic Risks to Humans volume 17 (Paris: International Agency for Research on Cancer), volume 40 (1986) cited in https://davidsuzuki.org/queen-of-green/dirty-dozen-bha-bht/
4. Study on Enhancing the Endocrine Disrupter Priority List with a Focus on Low Production Volume Chemicals, Revised Report to DG Environment (Hersholm, Denmark: DHI Water and Environment, 2007), http://ec.europa.eu/environment/endocrine/documents/final_report_2007.pdf cited in https://davidsuzuki.org/queen-of-green/dirty-dozen-bha-bht/

5. http://www.fda.gov/Cosmetics/ProductandIngredientSafety cited in https://davidsuzuki.org/queen-of-green/dirty-dozen-parabens/

6. DHI Water and Environment. Study on Enhancing the Endocrine Disrupter Priority List with a Focus on Low Production Volume Chemicals. Revised Report to DG Environment. Hersholm, Denmark: DHI, 2007. http://ec.europa.eu/environment/endocrine/documents/final_report_2007.pdf cited in https://davidsuzuki.org/queen-of-green/dirty-dozen-parabens/

7. https://onlinelibrary.wiley.com/doi/abs/10.1002/jat.1786

8. Handa, O. Kokura, S. et al. (2006) "Methylparaben potentiates UV-induced damage of skin keratinocytes" *Toxicology*. 227: 62-72 cited in https://davidsuzuki.org/queen-of-green/dirty-dozen-parabens/

9. Black, R. Hurley, F. and Havery, D. (2001) "Occurrence of 1,4-dioxane in cosmetic raw materials and finished cosmetic products" *Journal of AOAC International*. 84 (3): 666-670 cited in https://davidsuzuki.org/queen-of-green/dirty-dozen-sodium-laureth-sulfate/

10. https://www.cancer.org/cancer/cancer-causes/general-info/known-and-probable-human-carcinogens.html

11. Brashear, A. Unverzagt, F. et al. (1996) "Ethylene oxide neurotoxicity: a cluster of 12 nurses with peripheral and central nervous system toxicity" *Neurology*. 46 (4): 992-998 cited in https://davidsuzuki.org/queen-of-green/dirty-dozen-sodium-laureth-sulfate/

12. California. EPA. Office of Environmental Health Hazard Assessment. Chemicals Known to the State to Cause Cancer or Reproductive Toxicity. February 5, 2010. http://www.oehha.org/prop65/prop65_list/files/P65single020510.pdf cited in https://davidsuzuki.org/queen-of-green/dirty-dozen-sodium-laureth-sulfate/

13. https://www.cancer.org/cancer/cancer-causes/general-info/known-and-probable-human-carcinogens.html

14. https://www.ncbi.nlm.nih.gov/pubmed/27096631

15. https://onlinelibrary.wiley.com/doi/pdf/10.1002/3527600418.mb10846e0020 https://www.choice.com.au/health-and-body/beauty-and-personal-care/skin-care-and-cosmetics/articles/chemicals-in-cosmetics

16. https://www.ncbi.nlm.nih.gov/pubmed/12571683

17. Survey of liquid hand soaps, including health and environmental assessments, Survey of chemical substances in consumer products (Danish EPA, 2006), no. 69 cited in https://davidsuzuki.org/wp-content/uploads/2017/10/dirty-dozen-cosmetics-ingredients-backgrounder.pdf

REFERENCES AND RESOURCES

18. https://www.icac.org/seep/documents/reports/2010_interpretative_summary.pdf

19. https://www.ncbi.nlm.nih.gov/pubmed/11392380

20. http://www.who.int/mediacentre/factsheets/fs225/en/

21. http://time.com/4422774/tampons-toxic-cancer/

22. https://ehjournal.biomedcentral.com/articles/10.1186/s12940-015-0043-6

21. http://time.com/4422774/tampons-toxic-cancer/

22. https://ehjournal.biomedcentral.com/articles/10.1186/s12940-015-0043-6

Courageously beautiful

1. Reinhold Niebuhr

2. Johann Wolfgang von Goethe

General references/books that have influenced my work, not already listed above

Robbins, T. (1992) *Awaken the Giant Within*. London: Simon & Schuster.

Roth, G. (2009) *Women, Food and God*. New York: Scribner.

Roth, G. (2011) *Lost and Found: Unexpected Revelations About Food and Money*. New York: Viking Penguin.

Live speakers who have influenced my work

Marianne Williamson

Dr John Demartini

Tony Robbins

If you need support for an eating disorder, you might like to contact a counsellor or psychologist in your area. Organisations that offer support include The Butterfly Foundation in Australia: www.butterflyfoundation.org.au They also have a hotline that you can phone to speak to someone who can help you. You can call their national (AU) help line on 1800334673. You can also chat online or email them. In New Zealand, you might like to reach out to EDANZ at www.ed.org.nz who can best direct you to support in your local area.

notes